# The Herbal Beverage Book

## Simple and Delicious Recipes for the Whole Family

Robin Belliveau

Practical Intuitive Media LLC

ISBN-13: 978-0-578-72439-3 Paperback


LIBRARY OF CONGRESS CATALOG
Identifier: LCCN 2020912614

Published in the United States of America by
Practical Intuitive Media LLC
Worcester, Massachusetts, USA


www.robinbelliveau.com

Book design by Robin Belliveau
Updated Edition, September 2020

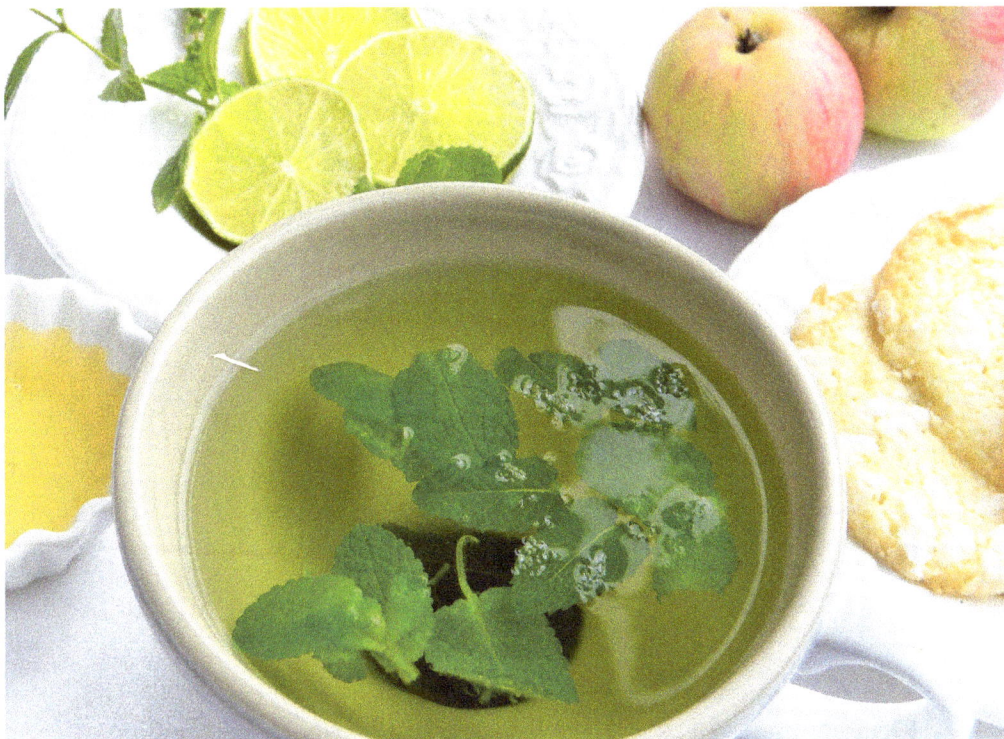

*"Let food be thy medicine and medicine be thy food."*

*Hippocrates, 400 B.C.*

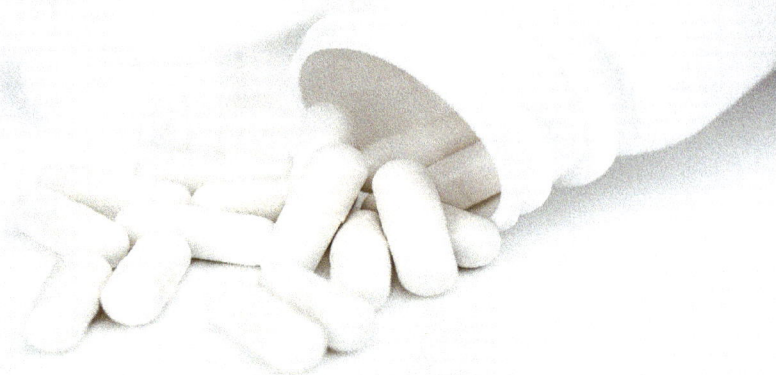

## Dietary and Herbal Supplements

Federal law defines dietary supplements as products that:
• You take by mouth (such as a tablet, capsule, powder, or liquid)
• Are made to supplement the diet
• Have one or more dietary ingredients, including vitamins, minerals, herbs or other botanicals, amino acids, enzymes, tissues from organs or glands, or extracts of these
• Are labeled as being dietary supplements.

Herbal supplements—sometimes called botanicals—are a type of dietary supplement containing one or more herbs.

The amount of scientific evidence on dietary supplements varies widely—there is a lot of information on some and very little on others. If you're considering using a dietary supplement, it's important to keep the following in mind:

• Supplements you buy from stores or online may differ in important ways from products tested in research studies.
• Dietary supplements may interact with your medications or pose risks if you have certain medical problems or are going to have surgery.
• Many dietary supplements haven't been tested in pregnant women, nursing mothers, or children.
• What's listed on the label of a dietary supplement may not be what's in the product. For example, some products marketed for weight loss, sexual enhancement, or bodybuilding have been found to contain prescription drugs not allowed in dietary supplements or other ingredients not listed on the label, and some of these ingredients may be unsafe.
• Rules for manufacturing and distributing dietary supplements are less strict than those for prescription or over-the-counter drugs. Although the U.S. Food and Drug Administration (FDA) requires that companies submit safety data about any new ingredient not sold in the United States in a dietary supplement before 1994, the FDA is not authorized to review dietary supplements for safety and effectiveness before they are marketed.

NCCIH has provided this material for your information. It is not intended to substitute for the medical expertise and advice of your health care provider(s). We encourage you to discuss any decisions about treatment or care with your health care provider. The mention of any product, service, or therapy is not an endorsement by NCCIH.

(Last Updated: February 2020)

# Table of Contents

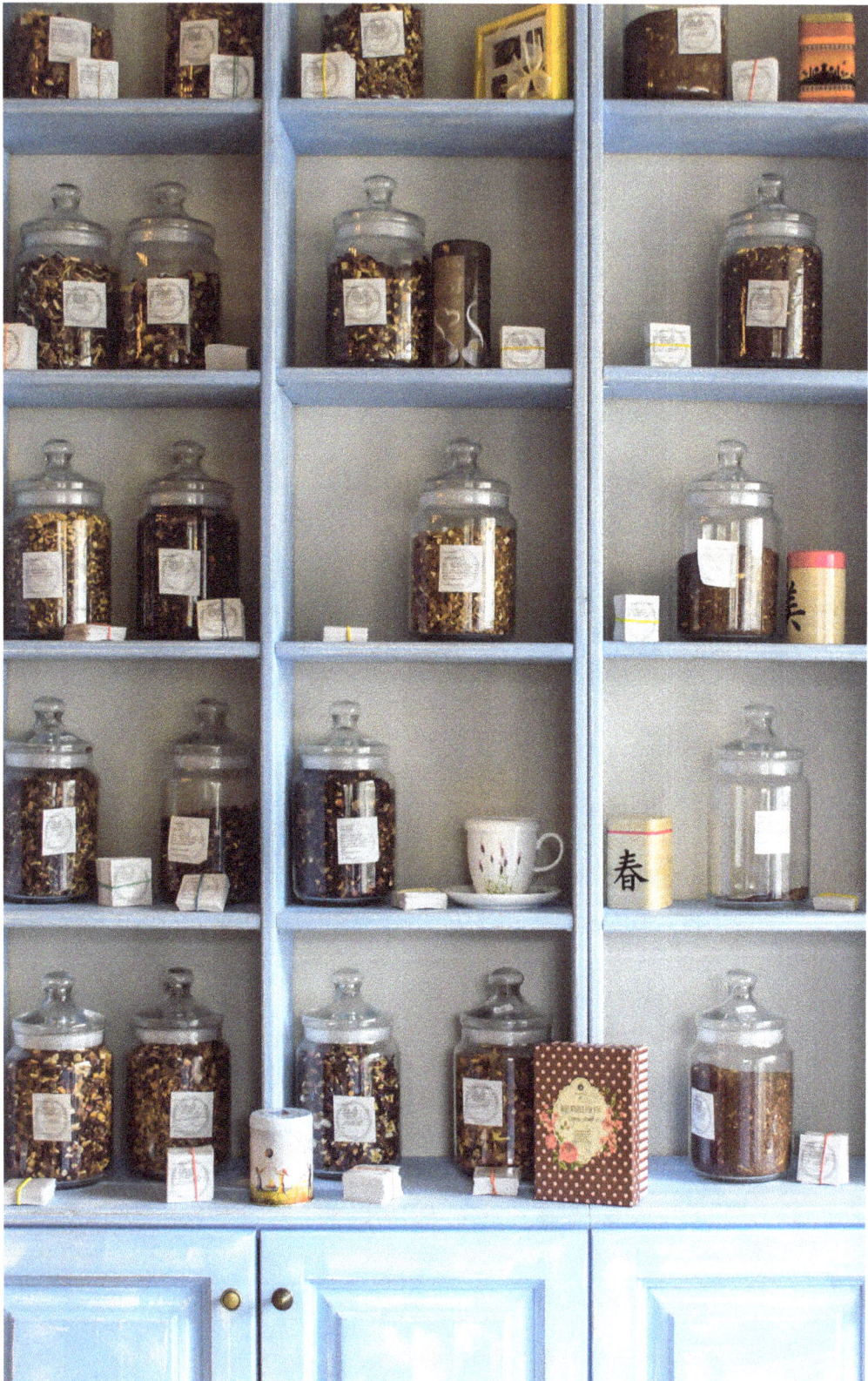

# Introduction

While searching for great tasting drinks for my children which didn't have either a lot of food coloring, sugar, or both, I stumbled into the world of making my own herbal beverages. None of my children liked the traditional black teas you find at the grocery store, so I was on a quest to find healthy alternatives. When I looked at the prepackaged herbal teas, I saw that the teas averaged twenty five dollars per pound. I also didn't like that some of the herbs were on the bitter side, so in order to make them taste good, you had to add a lot of sweetener.

After some research, and a lot of experimenting with different combinations, I was able to come up with herbal recipes that are very kid friendly as far as taste but also had the bonus of having great overall health benefits. The recipes in this book are kid-tested, easy to make, and affordable.

When trying the recipes yourself, pay attention to how each of them makes you feel, especially if you are using them to relieve the symptoms of a specific ailment. For example, if one recipe for a cough doesn't seem to do much for you, try one of the others.

In the back of the book, I put together an index of the herbs used in the recipes with a concise description of what each have been traditionally used for. I urge you to not only try the recipes that I have put together for you, but also try some of the herbs in teas by themselves.

I hope your education about herbs does not stop with the recipes and information included here. There are many more herbs available to you. I encourage you to do some further reading about them from other sources, such as the ones included in the back of this book.

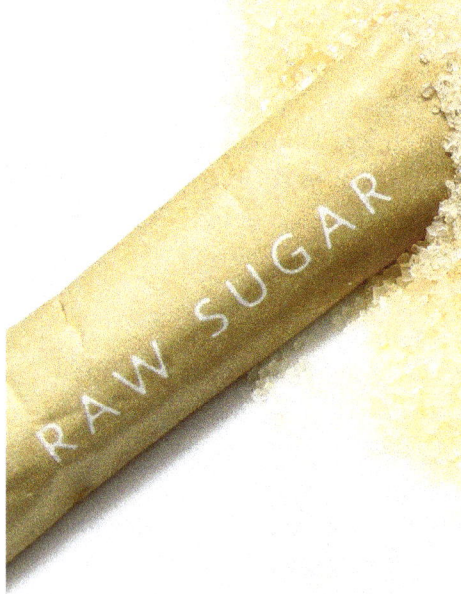

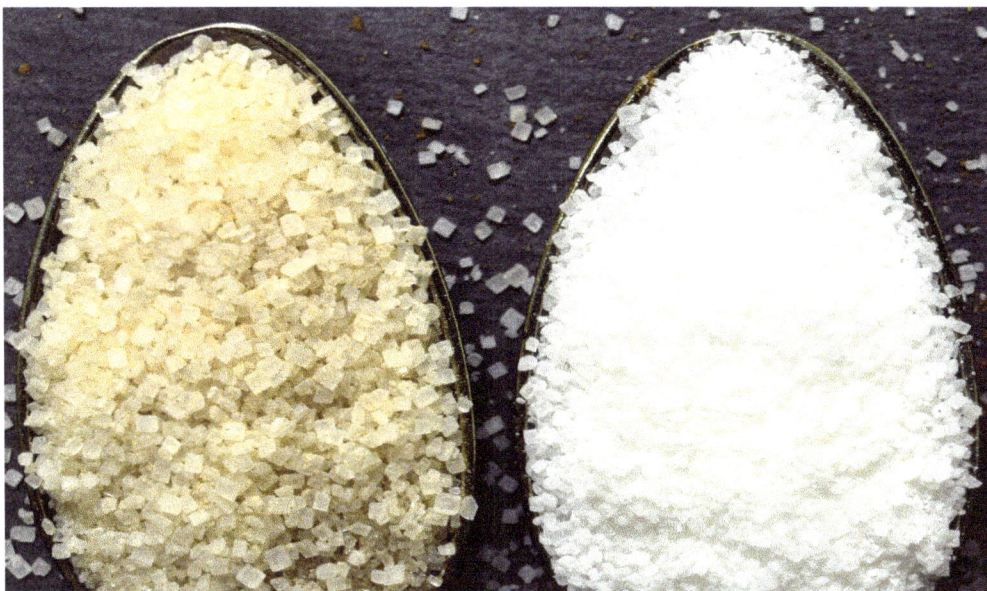

# A Note About Sweeteners

I would advise tasting all of the beverage recipes without sweetener, aside from the lemonades and syrups, so you can get a sense of how much sweetener you may need. You will find that many of them may not need to be sweetened at all. If you would like to omit processed sugar for health reasons, try alternatives such as raw honey, one hundred percent fruit juice, coconut sugar, maple sugar, xylitol, stevia, or agave. Experiment with the ones you like. Just as some juices are sweeter than others, some of the extracted sugars have different sweetnesses and aftertastes as well.

As far as stevia goes, a lot of the prepackaged stevia on the market has fillers or other sweeteners such as fiber or xylitol so look very closely at the ingredients. Use the prepackaged stevia according to the package directions, although you often need a lot less than they recommend. It does have a slightly bitter aftertaste and I have heard of anecdotal allergic reactions, so keep this in mind if you use it.

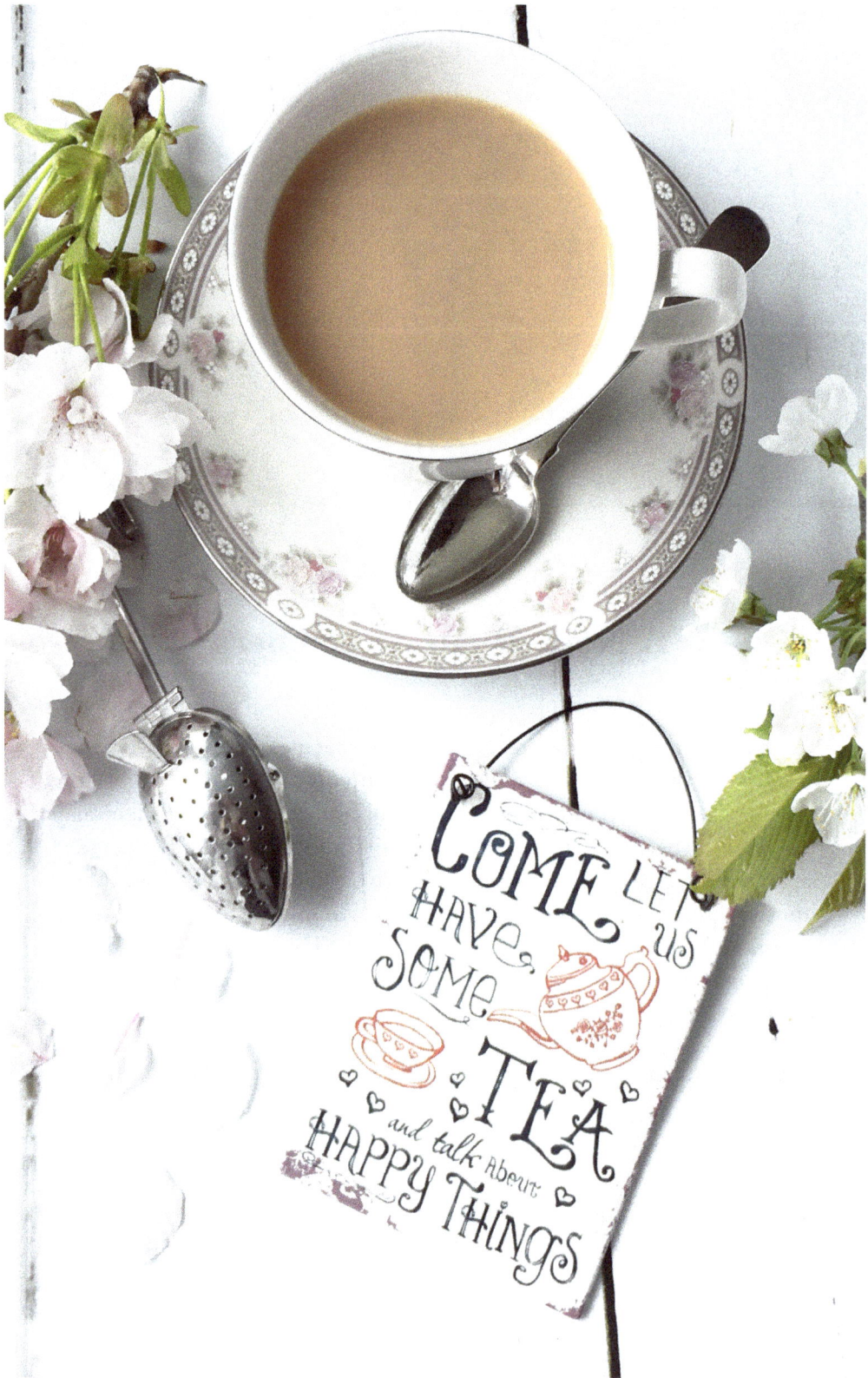

# Herbal Teas

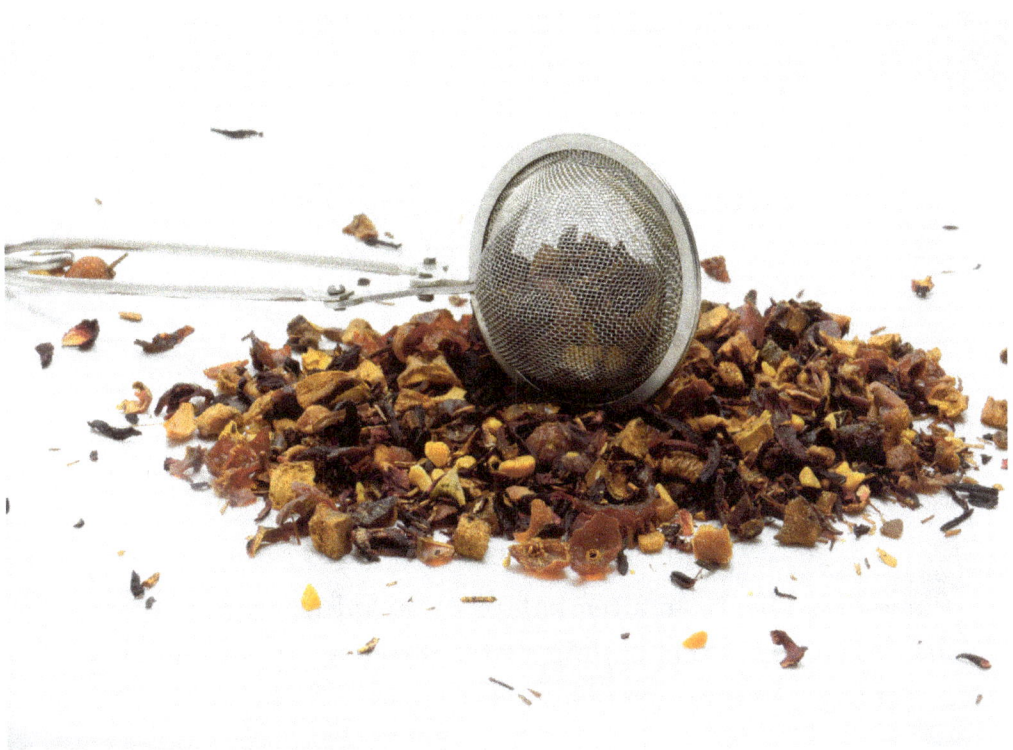

The longer you let the herbs brew, the more of the properties you can extract from them. Some herbs get sweeter the longer you let them steep as well. However, you may want to start on the weaker side for herbs that you may not be familiar with. I listed these teas by typical symptom relief but they can be enjoyed at any time.

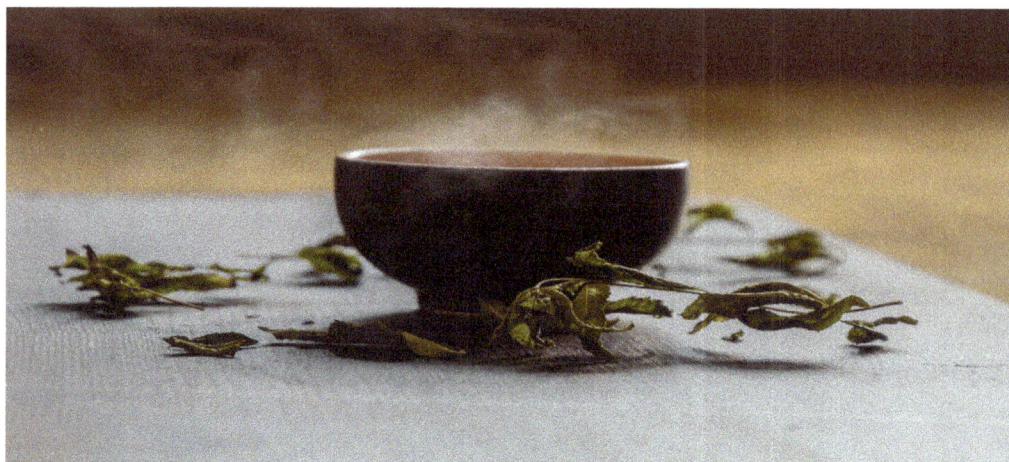

# Immunity Boosting Tea

~ immunity, illness and recovery

1 tsp dried elderberries
1 tsp dried lemon balm
1 tsp dried nettles
1 tsp dried rose hips

Place dried herbs in a tea ball or other infuser and place inside tea cup. Pour boiling water into tea cup and let sit for at least 10 minutes. Sweeten to taste.

Mix the herbs into a large jar to store in your cabinet to have on hand before cold and flu season starts. It not only helps with prevention but also aids in getting over illnesses and general symptom relief.

This is a great tea to give as a gift.

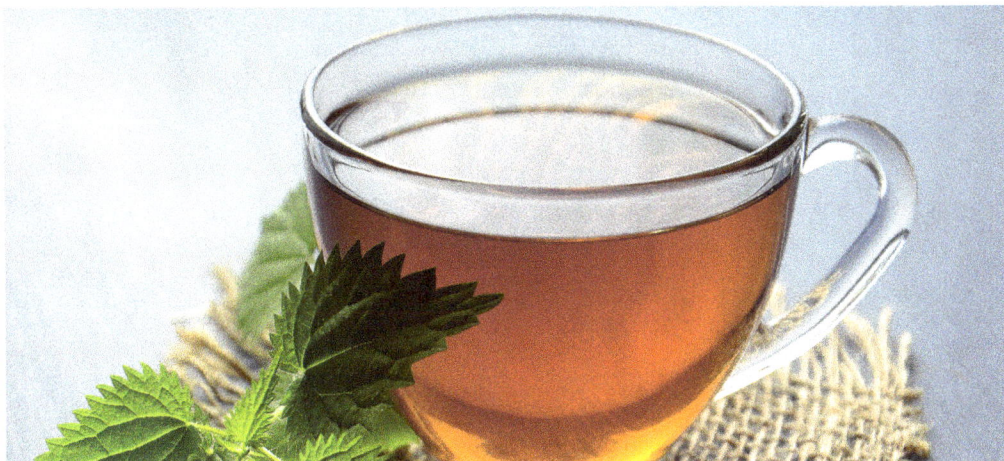

# Nourishing Tea
~ allergies, recovery, leg cramps

1 tsp dried nettles
1 tsp dried oatstraw
1 tsp dried alfalfa

Place dried herbs in a tea ball or other infuser and place inside tea cup. Pour boiling water into tea cup and let sit for at least 5 minutes. Sweeten to taste.

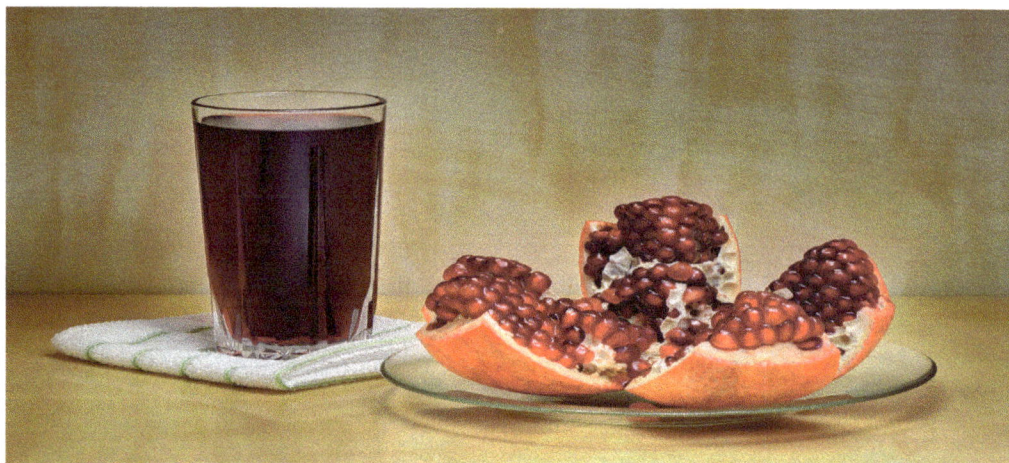

# Soothing Tea
~ anxiety, sleeplessness

    1 tsp dried catnip leaves
    2 tsp dried chamomile flowers
    splash of pomegranate juice *
        (or other fruit juice)

Place dried herbs in a tea ball or other infuser and place inside tea cup. Pour boiling water into tea cup and let sit for at least 5 minutes. Add pomegranate or other fruit juice.  Sweeten to taste.

*Catnip has a very strong taste and the juice counteracts this.

Chamomile and catnip both tend to have a diuretic affect so you may not want to serve this too close to bed time.

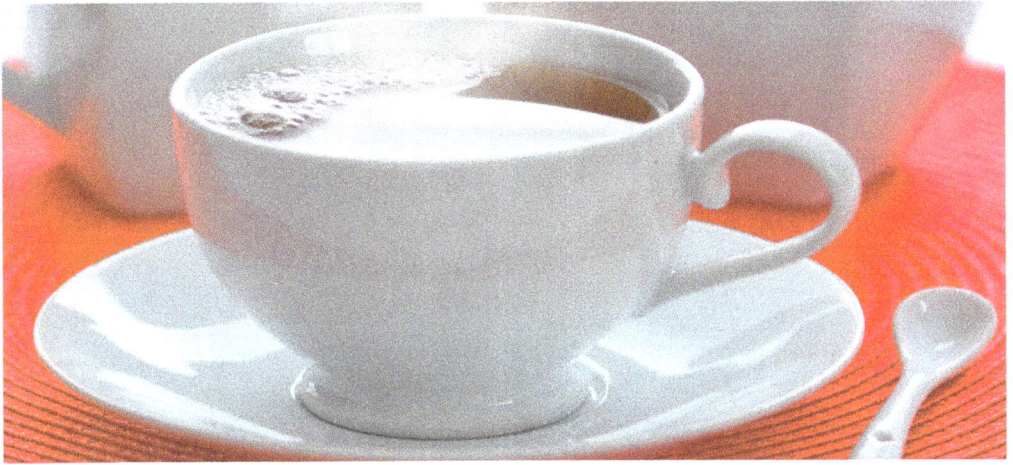

# Headache Tea
~ headache, stress

1 tsp dried chamomile flowers
1 tsp dried spearmint leaves
1 tsp dried lemon balm

Place dried herbs in a tea ball or other infuser and place inside tea cup. Pour boiling water into tea cup and let sit for at least 5 minutes. Sweeten to taste.

Chamomile tends to have a diuretic affect so you may not want to serve this too close to bed time.

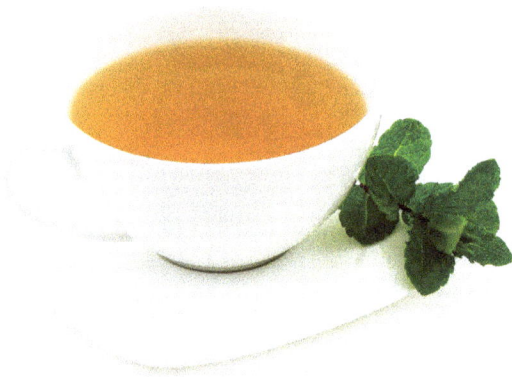

# Anti-Anxiety Tea

~ anxiety, stress

1 tsp dried catnip
1 tsp dried licorice root*
1 tsp dried lemon balm

Place dried herbs in a tea ball or other infuser and place inside tea cup. Pour boiling water into tea cup and let sit for at least 5 minutes. Sweeten to taste.

Catnip tends to have a diuretic affect so you may not want to serve this too close to bed time.

* Please consult your herbal supplier for health warnings regarding licorice root. It is not for prolonged use. If for any reason you can't use licorice root, substitute it in this recipe with 1 tsp dried spearmint leaves.

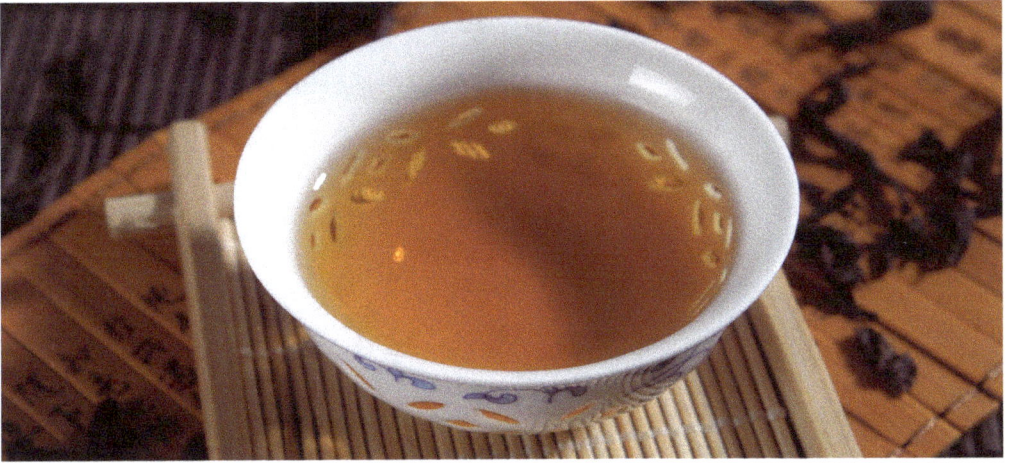

# Growing Pains Tea

~ leg cramps, growing pains

1 tsp dried nettles
1 tsp dried marshmallow root
1 tsp dried oatstraw


Place dried herbs in a tea ball or other infuser and place inside tea cup. Pour boiling water into tea cup and let sit for at least 5 minutes. Sweeten to taste.

May also help with hay fever.

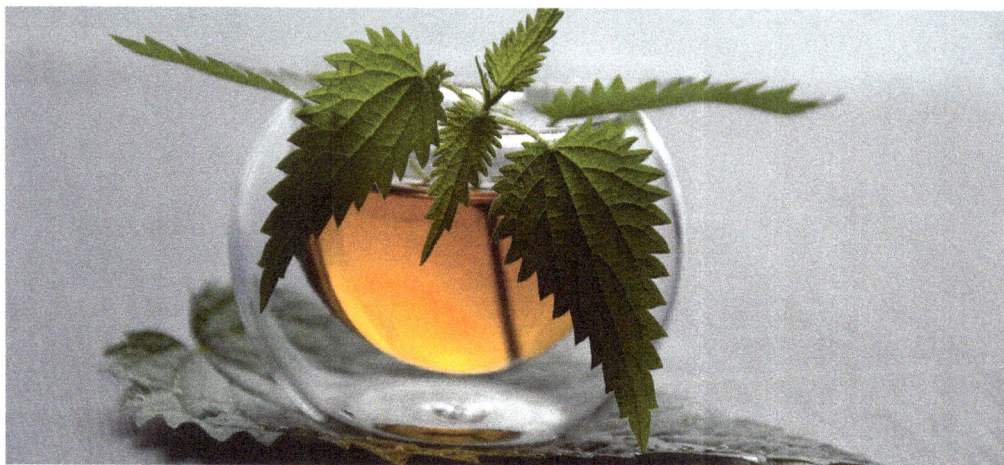

# Allergy Tea
~ allergies, recovery

1 tsp dried nettles
1 tsp dried oatstraw
1/2 tsp dried licorice root*


Place dried herbs in a tea ball or other infuser and place inside tea cup. Pour boiling water into tea cup and let sit for at least 5 minutes. Sweeten to taste.

* Please consult your herbal supplier for health warnings regarding licorice root. It is not for prolonged use. If for any reason you can't use licorice root, substitute it in this recipe with 1 tsp dried spearmint leaves.

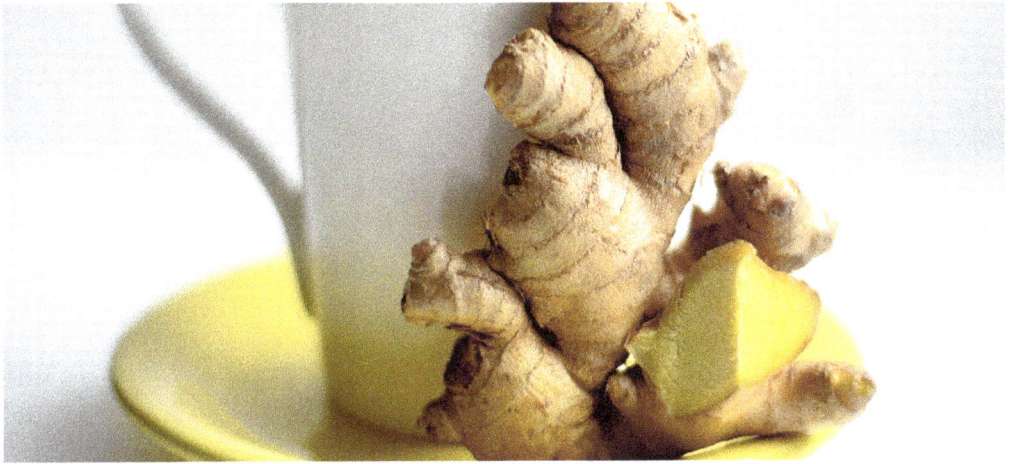

# Anti-Nausea Tea
~ stomach complaints, stress

1 tsp dried chamomile flowers
1/2 tsp dried (or minced fresh) ginger root
1 tsp dried lemon balm

Place dried herbs in a tea ball or other infuser and place inside tea cup. Pour boiling water into tea cup and let sit for 3 to 5 minutes. Sweeten to taste.

Chamomile tends to have a diuretic affect so you may not want to drink this too close to bed time.

May also help with headache, constipation or heartburn.

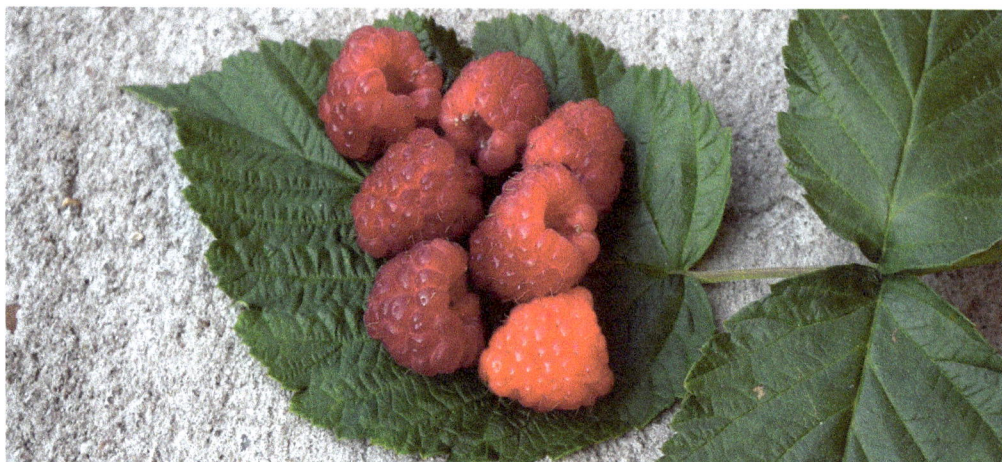

# Diarrhea Relief Tea
~ diarrhea, sore throat

2 tsp dried red raspberry leaf
1 tsp dried chamomile flowers

Place dried herbs in a tea ball or other infuser and place inside tea cup. Pour boiling water into tea cup and let sit for at least 10 minutes. Sweeten to taste.

Chamomile tends to have a diuretic affect so you may not want to serve this too close to bed time.

May also help with sore throats and any mouth issues such as canker sores or other mouth irritations.

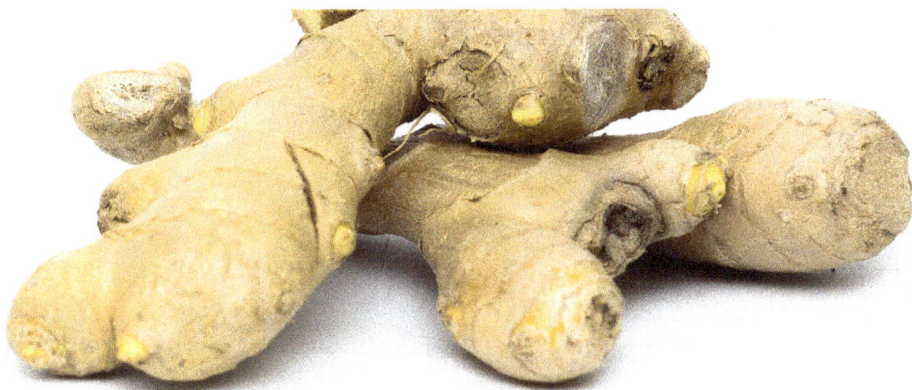

# Cooling Stomach Tea
~ stomach complaints, heartburn

1/2 tsp dried (or minced fresh) ginger root
1 tsp dried red raspberry leaf


Place dried herbs in a tea ball or other infuser and place inside tea cup. Pour boiling water into tea cup and let sit for at least 5 minutes. Sweeten to taste.

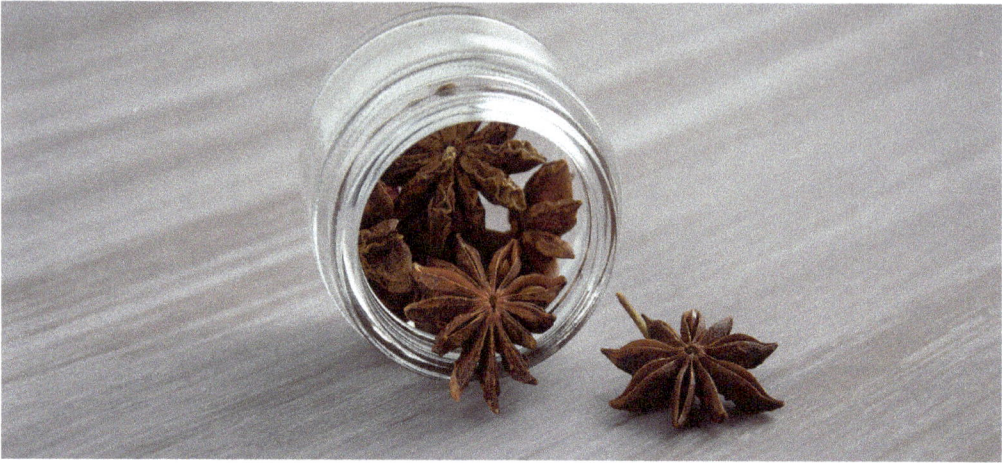

# Warming Stomach Tea
~ upset stomach, constipation

1 tsp fennel seeds
1 tsp anise seeds
2 tsp dried chamomile flowers


Place dried herbs in a tea ball or other infuser and place inside tea cup. Pour boiling water into tea cup and let sit for at least 5 minutes. Sweeten to taste.

Chamomile tends to have a diuretic affect so you may not want to serve this too close to bed time.

This tea is great for any stomach complaints but is especially good for gas or bloating.

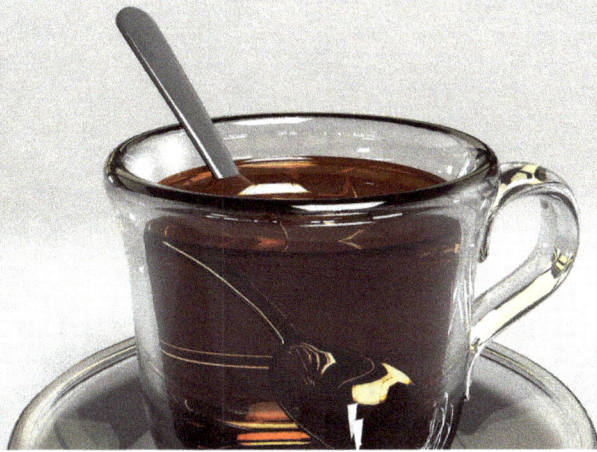

# Throat Tea
~ sore throat, mouth irritations

1 tsp dried marshmallow root
1 tsp dried red raspberry leaf
1/2 tsp dried licorice root*

Place dried herbs in a tea ball or other infuser and place inside tea cup. Pour boiling water into tea cup and let sit for 10 minutes. Sweeten to taste.

* Please consult your herbal supplier for health warnings regarding licorice root. It is not for prolonged use. If for any reason you can't use licorice root, substitute it in this recipe with 1 tsp dried spearmint leaves.

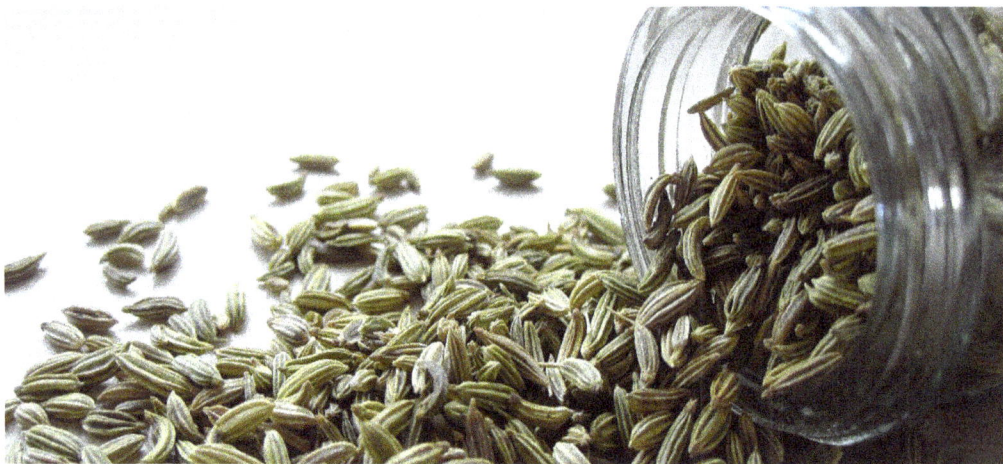

# Cough Relief Tea
~ cough suppressing

1/2 tsp wild cherry bark
1 tsp dried licorice root*
1/2 tsp fennel seed
1 tsp dried chamomile flowers

Place dried herbs in a tea ball or other infuser and place inside tea cup. Pour boiling water into tea cup and let sit for 10 minutes. Sweeten to taste.

Chamomile tends to have a diuretic affect so you may not want to serve this too close to bed time.

* Please consult your herbal supplier for health warnings regarding licorice root. It is not for prolonged use. If for any reason you can't use licorice root, substitute it in this recipe with 1 tsp dried spearmint leaves.

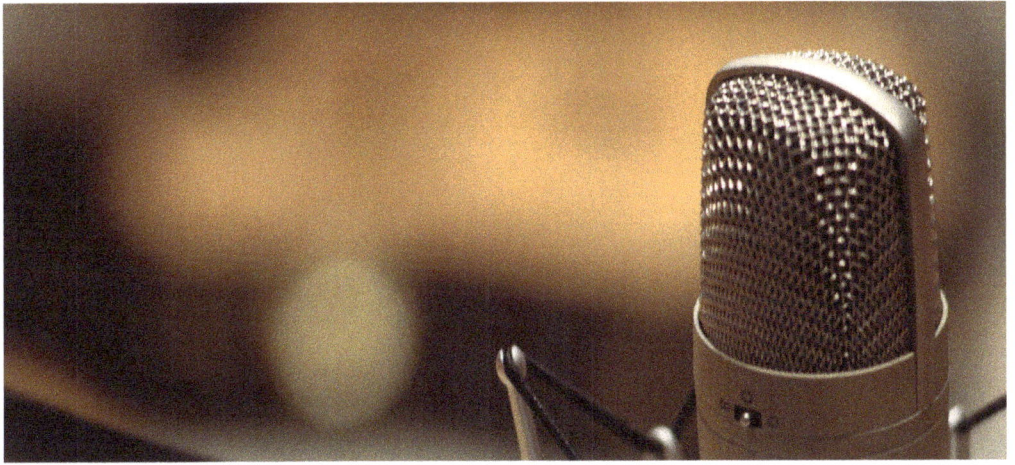

# Singer's Tea
~ sore throat

1/2 tsp dried licorice root*

Place dried herbs in a tea ball or other infuser and place inside tea cup. Pour boiling water into tea cup and let sit for 10 minutes. Licorice root is great for lubricating the vocal chords.

* Please consult your herbal supplier for health warnings regarding licorice root. It is not for prolonged use.

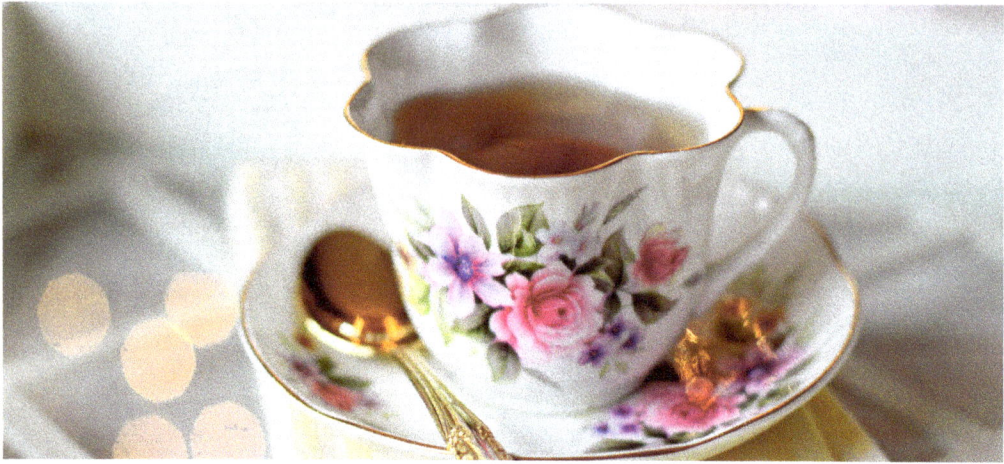

# Expectorant Tea
~ cough expectorant, sinus relief

2 tsp fennel seeds

Place fennel seeds in a tea ball or other infuser and place inside tea cup. Pour boiling water into tea cup and let sit for at least 5 minutes. Sweeten to taste.

This simple tea works amazingly well!

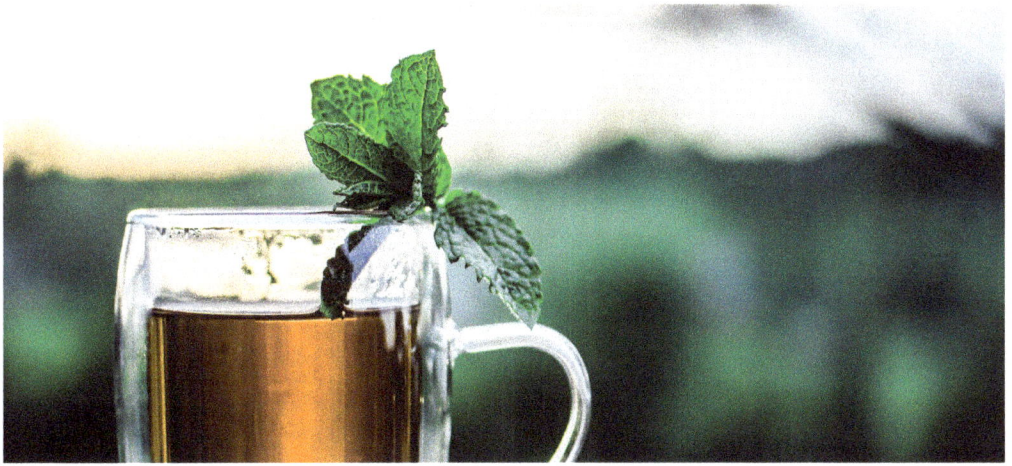

# Dry Cough Tea
~ cough suppressing and expectorant

1 tsp dried mullein
1 tsp dried marshmallow root
1/2 tsp dried spearmint leaves

Place dried herbs in a tea ball or other infusers and place inside tea cup. Pour boiling water into tea cup and let sit for at least 5 minutes. The longer you let it steep, the stronger the properties, and taste. Sweeten to taste.

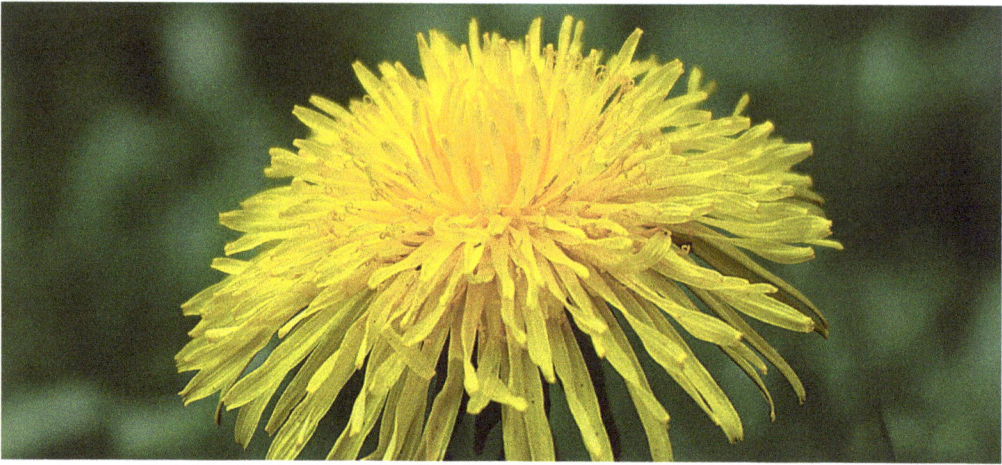

# Skin Clear Tea
~ acne, indigestion

1 tsp dried nettles
1 tsp dried calendula flowers
1/2 tsp dried dandelion root

Place dried herbs in a tea ball or other infuser and place inside tea cup. Pour boiling water into tea cup and let sit for 5 minutes. Sweeten to taste.

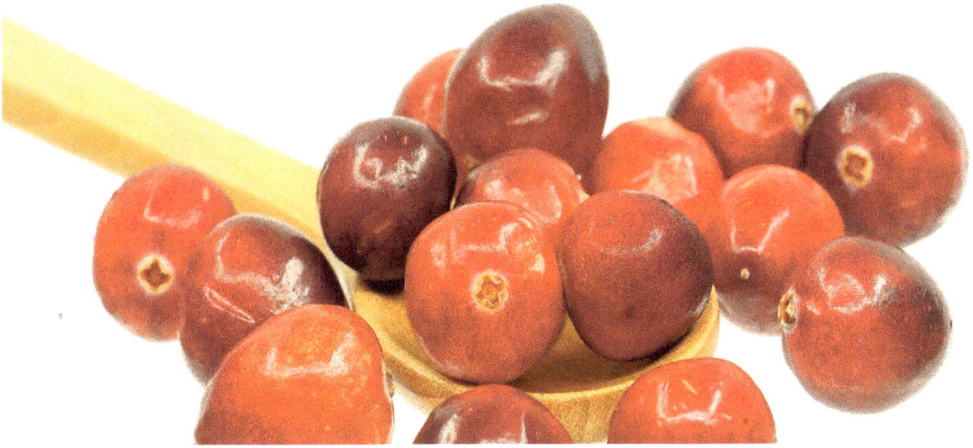

# Bladder Relief Tea
~ urinary discomfort

1 tsp dried marshmallow root
1 tsp dried nettles
1/2 cup 100% cranberry juice

Place dried herbs in a tea ball or other infuser and place inside tea cup. Pour boiling water into tea cup, about 1/2 full, and let sit for at least 10 minutes. Add cranberry juice. This cranberry juice is very sour so you may want to sweeten or use cranberry juice that is sweetened with another fruit juice.

This works very quickly at the first signs of any bladder discomfort. Keep drinking it until you notice is clearing up. It should help within a few hours. If symptoms don't improve within a day, or are severe, consult your health care professional immediately.

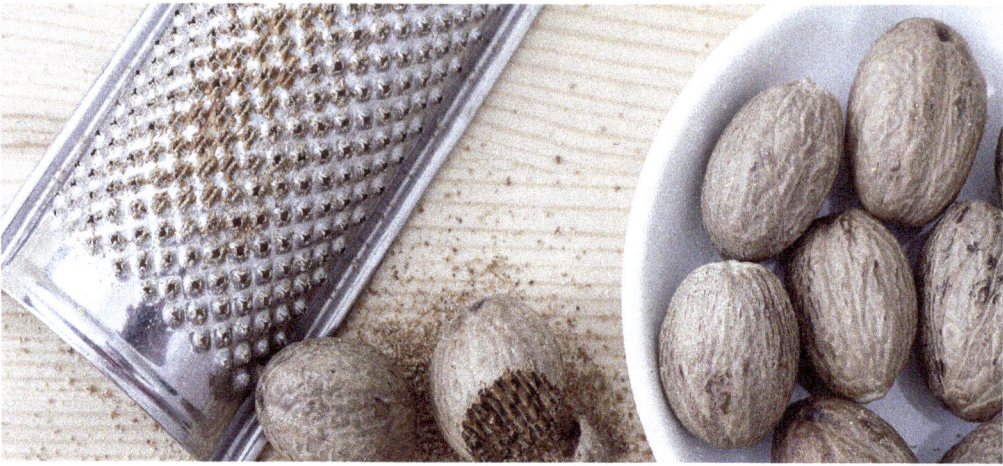

# Chai Tea
~ no caffeine, also great for digestion

1 tsp rooibos tea
1 whole clove
1/4 cinnamon stick
1/8 tsp dried ginger root
1 whole cardamom pod - broken
1/8 tsp ground nutmeg
sweetener - to taste
milk, or non-dairy alternative (if desired)


Place dried herbs in a tea ball or other infuser and place inside tea cup. Pour boiling water into tea cup and let sit for at least 5 minutes. Add sweetener and milk to taste.

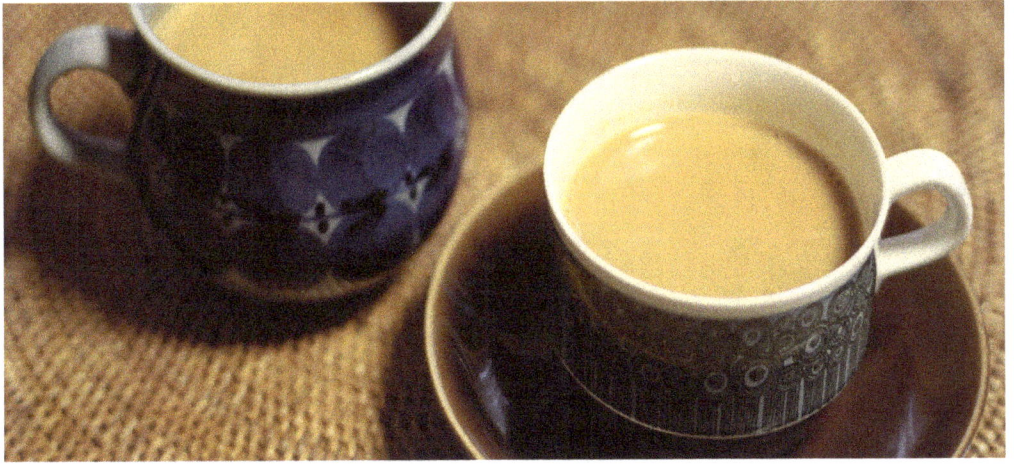

# Chocolate Chai

Add 1 tsp Chocolate Syrup (page 94)

# Vanilla Chai

Add 1 tsp Vanilla Syrup (page 96)

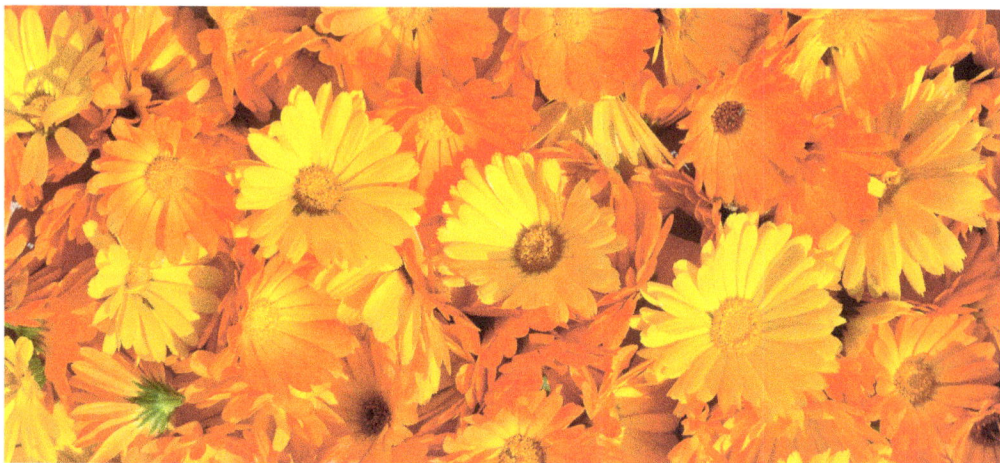

# Feel Better Tea
~ post illness recovery

1 tsp dried calendula flowers
1 tsp dried catnip
1 tsp dried spearmint leaves

Place dried herbs in a tea ball or other infuser and place inside tea cup. Pour boiling water into tea cup and let sit for at least 5 minutes. Sweeten to taste.

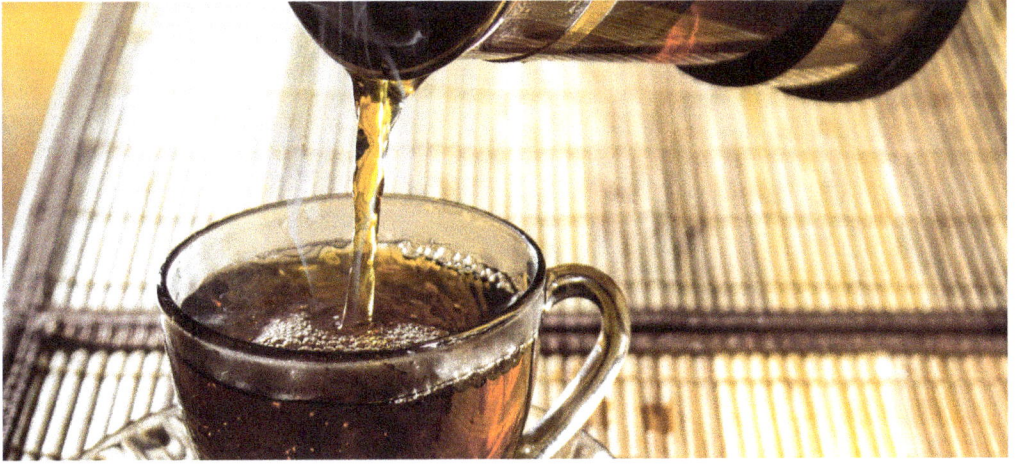

## Morning Cup of Tea
~ replacement for coffee

1 tsp green tea (try the gunpowder variety!)
1 tsp dried nettles
1/2 tsp orange peel


Place ingredients in a tea ball or other infuser and place inside tea cup. Pour boiling water into tea cup and let sit for at least 10 minutes. Sweeten to taste.

Make a batch to have on hand to put in your French press!

# Broths

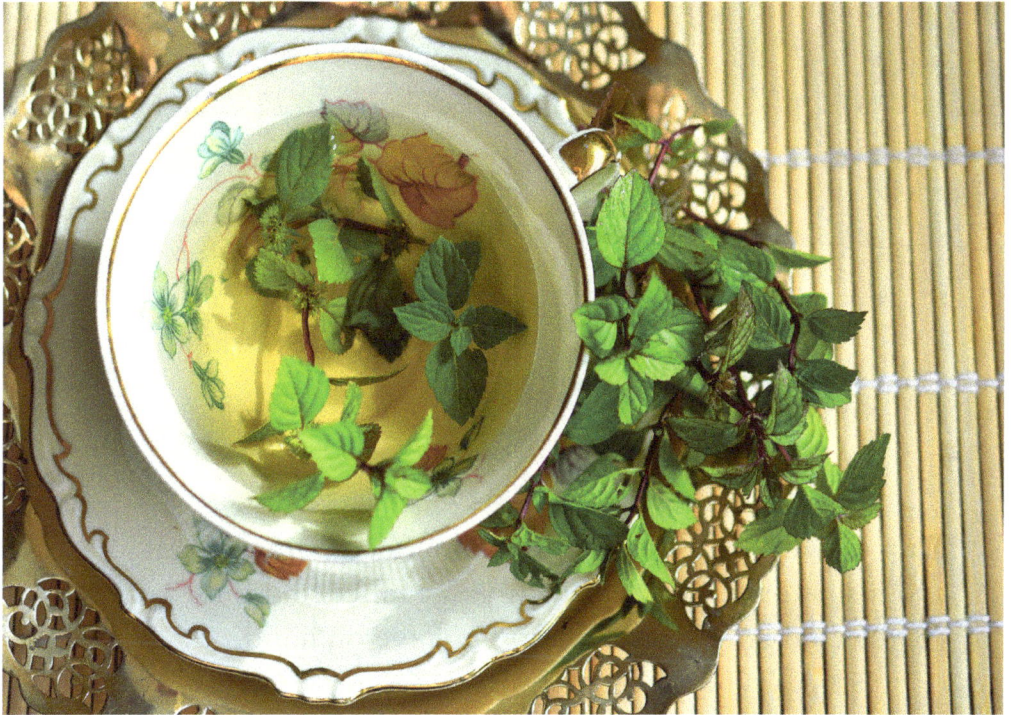

Broths are not only great during illnesses and for every day drinking during the cold winter months, but they are also great for adding different herbs to. If you aren't an herbal tea drinker, try these broths as an alternative.

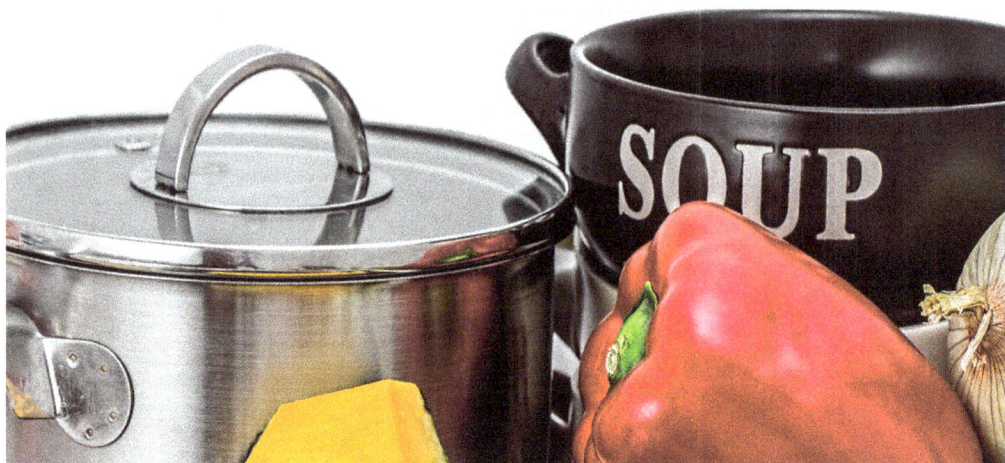

# Basic Broth

1 whole chicken (or 4 cups of vegetables)
1 tsp pink salt
crock pot or stock pot


Pink salt has many more trace minerals than table salt, and also more than sea salt. If you cannot find pink salt, you can substitute with what you have on hand.

Place chicken in crock pot and fill half way with water. Cover and cook on Low setting for 8 hours, or on High for 4 hours. The meat should be falling off the bones when it's done.

If you are vegetarian, you can make a broth using your favorite soup vegetables instead of the chicken. Cut the cook times in half.

Strain and store in the refrigerator.

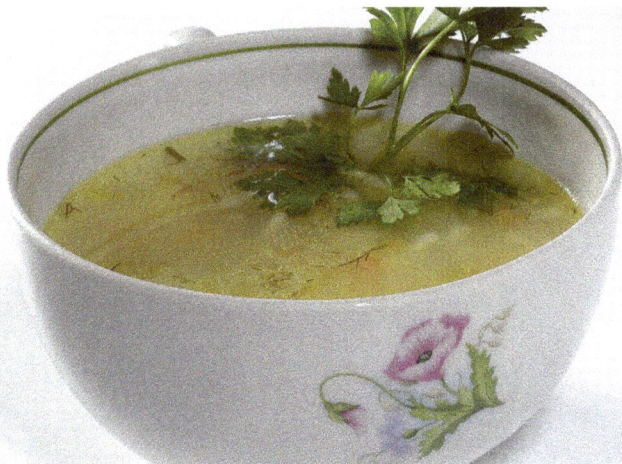

# Antiviral Broth 1

2 cups chicken or vegetable broth
1 clove garlic minced
2 tsp chopped onion
1 tsp rose hips
1/2 tsp astragalus root powder
        or 1/2 inch piece of dried astragalus root


Combine all ingredients in a medium saucepan. Heat to boiling. Reduce heat, cover and simmer for 10 minutes. Strain if desired and serve. For a hearty soup, add vegetables, noodles, or rice, to taste.

For added immune boosting or to help with congestion, add a dash of cayenne.

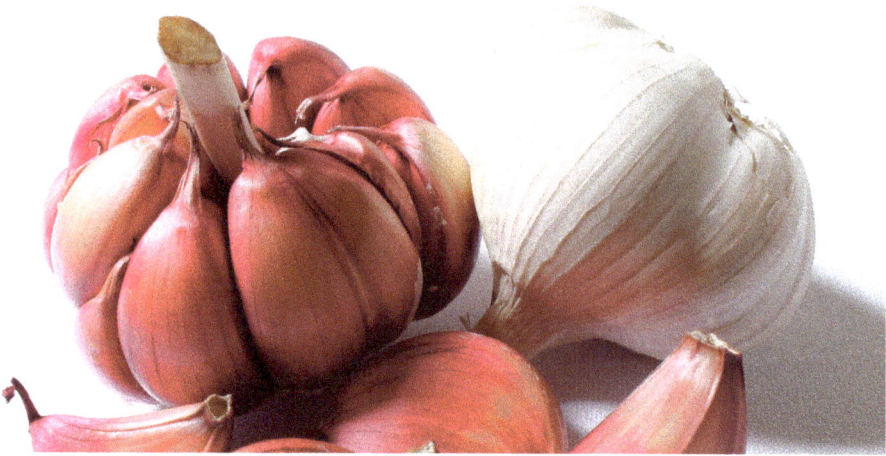

# Antiviral Broth 2

4 cups chicken or vegetable broth
2 cloves minced garlic
1/4 tsp dried rosemary, or 1 sprig fresh
1/4 tsp dried basil, or 1 tsp fresh
1/4 tsp dried lemon balm, or 1 tsp fresh
1/4 tsp dried nettles, or 1 tsp fresh

Combine all ingredients in a medium saucepan. Heat to boiling. Reduce heat, cover and simmer for 10 minutes. Strain and serve.

For added immune boosting or to help with congestion, add a dash of cayenne!

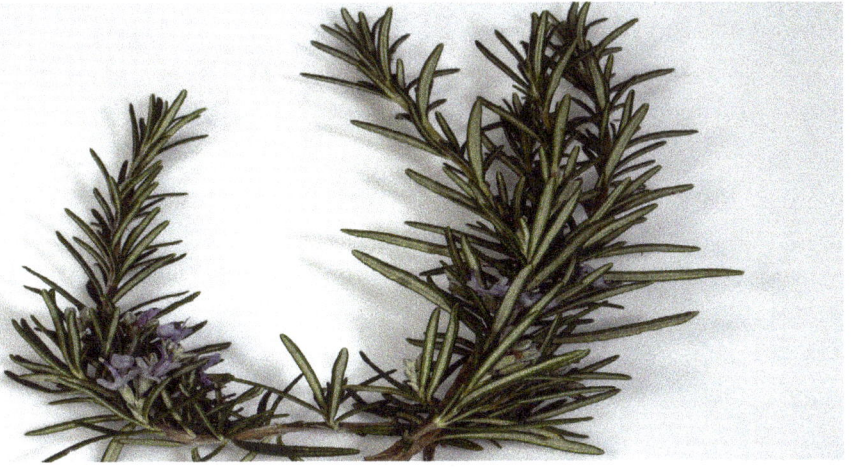

# Migraine Relief Broth

2 cups chicken or vegetable broth
1/2 tsp dried rosemary, or 1 sprig fresh


Combine all ingredients in a medium saucepan. Heat to boiling. Reduce heat, cover and simmer for 5 minutes or until rosemary is aromatic. Strain and serve.

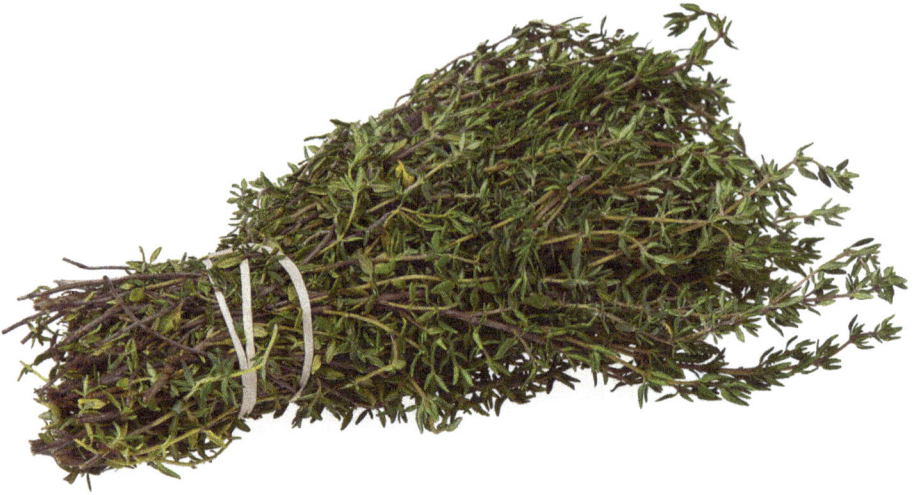

# Cough Relief Broth

2 cups chicken or vegetable broth
1 clove garlic minced
1/4 tsp dried thyme
1/4 tsp dried wild cherry bark
1/4 tsp dried mullein


Combine all ingredients in a medium saucepan. Heat to boiling. Reduce heat, cover and simmer for 10 minutes. Strain and serve.

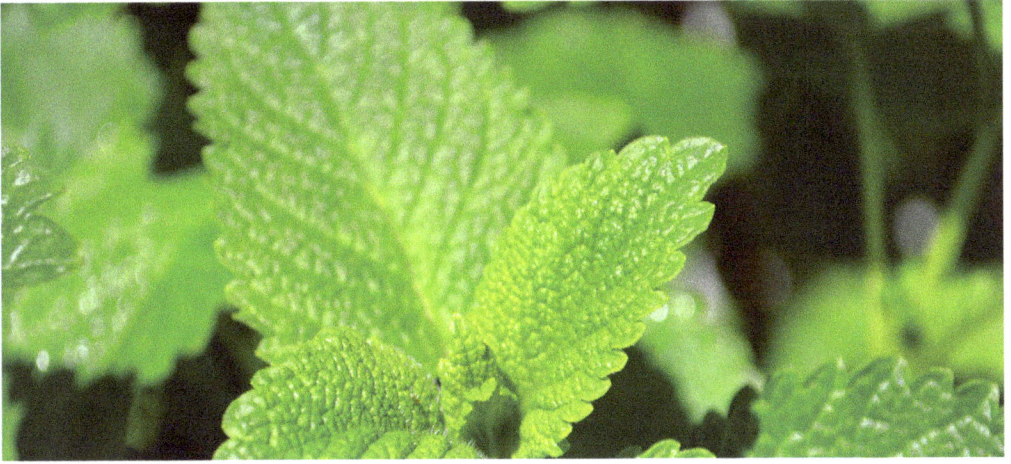

# Anti-Anxiety Broth

2 cups chicken or vegetable broth
1/4 tsp dried rosemary
1 tsp dried oatstraw
1 tsp dried lemon balm


Combine all ingredients in a medium saucepan. Heat to boiling. Reduce heat, cover and simmer for 10 minutes. Strain and serve.

# Milks

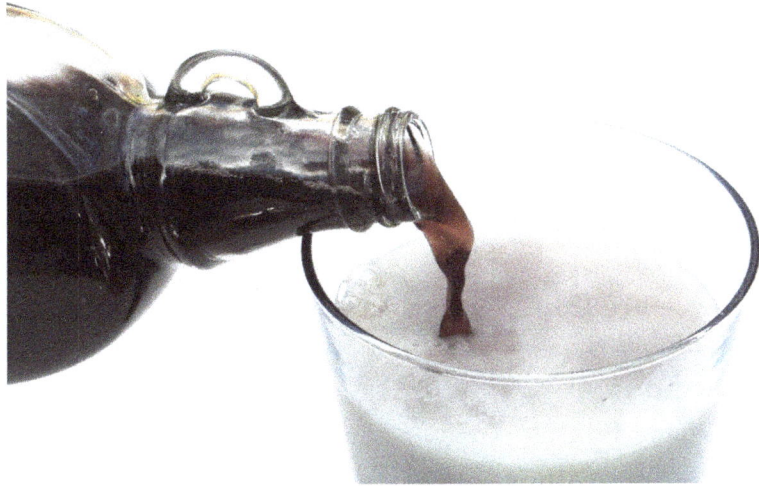

The following herbal milk recipes can be used with dairy milk or you can also use non-dairy options such as almond milk, coconut milk, hemp milk, soy milk, oat milk or rice milk. The beginning of this section has recipes for my favorite of those non-dairy alternatives, if you would like to make your own to store in the refrigerator. The following herbal milk recipes are for making warm milks which you may also chill.

Also refer to the syrup section starting on page 87 and try any of those syrups in your milk too.

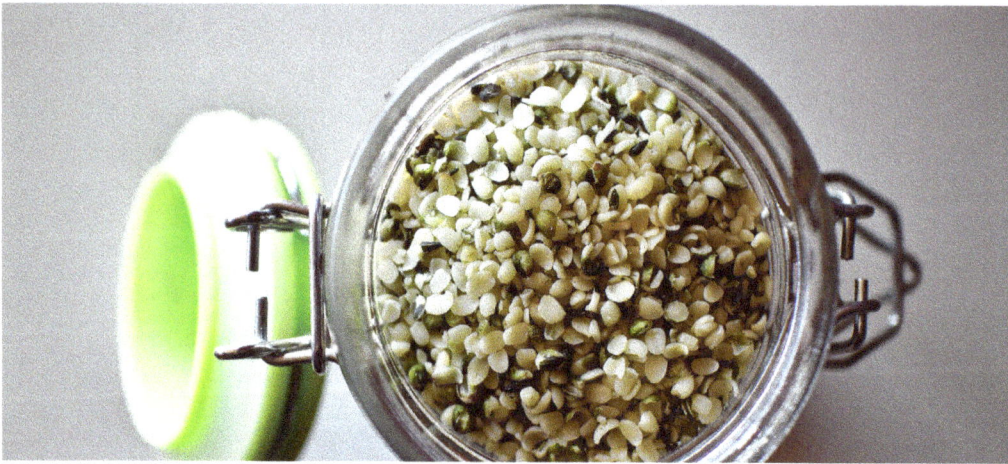

# Hemp Milk

1/3 cup raw shelled hemp seeds
6 cups water
1 Tbsp raw honey
     or 2 pitted dates (to sweeten, if desired)
nut milk bag or strainer - bag works best

Pour the water into the blender. Add hemp seeds and the honey or dates, if desired. Blend until frothy, no seeds can be seen, and it looks like milk. Strain into a large bowl using a nut bag or a fine mesh strainer. Using a canning or kitchen funnel, pour the milk into a pitcher and refrigerate.

It is not necessary to strain the milk but it tates a little less "nutty" if you do.

Use within 7 days.

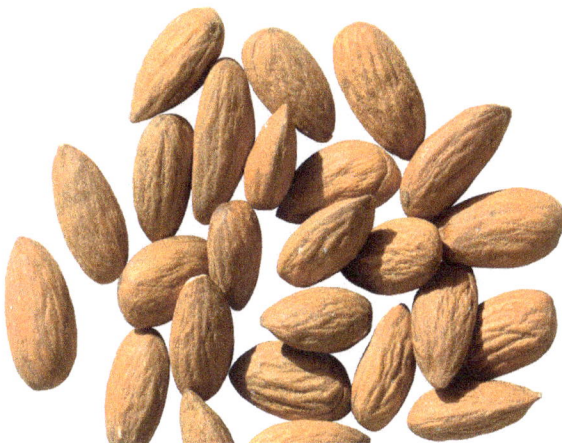

# Nut Milk

1/2 cup almonds, hazelnuts or coconut
6 cups water
nut milk bag or strainer - bag works best

Soaking the nuts before use is best, but in a pinch you can skip this step. Soaking removes phytic acid. I think it tastes better if you do soak them. To soak, put them in a bowl, cover them with water, let them sit on the kitchen counter for 4-6 hours, drain, and rinse. Remove the brown skins from the almonds if using them.

Fill the blender with the water. Add nuts and blend until frothy, no chunks can be seen and it looks like milk. Strain into a large bowl using a nut bag or a fine mesh strainer. Using a canning or kitchen funnel, pour the milk into a pitcher and refrigerate.

Use within 7 days.

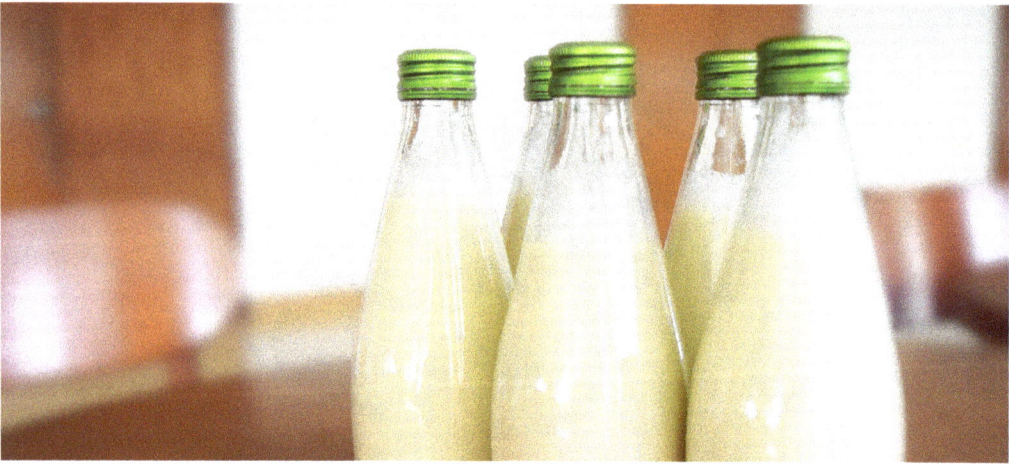

# Cough Milk 1

1 tsp dried mullein
1 tsp dried wild cherry bark
2 cups milk

Mix dried herbs and milk in a small saucepan. You may also place herbs in a tea ball so you don't have to strain them later. Heat on medium/low heat until steaming. Heat 5 minutes longer then remove from heat. Sweeten to taste. Strain, cool slightly and serve.

You may refrigerate before serving.

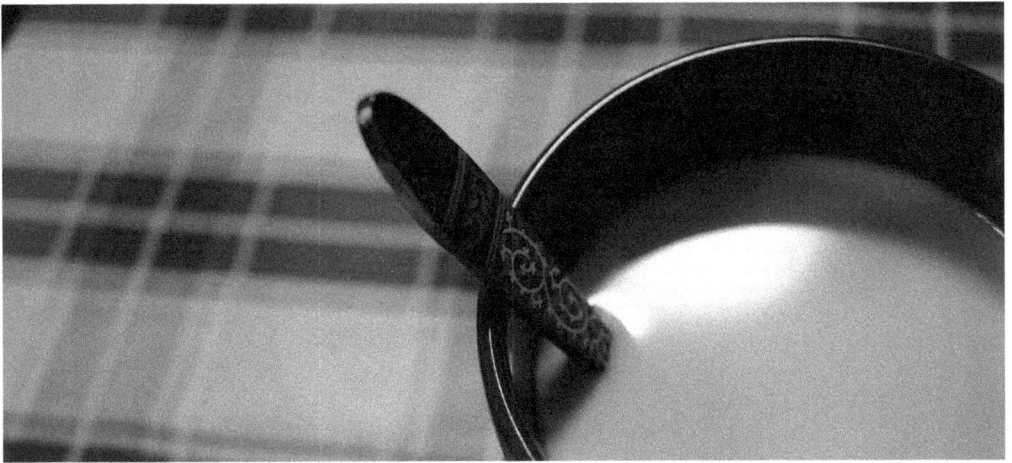

# Cough Milk 2

1 tsp dried licorice root*
1 tsp dried marshmallow root
2 cups milk

Mix dried herbs and milk in a small saucepan. You may also place herbs in a tea ball so you don't have to strain them later. Heat on medium/low heat until steaming. Heat 5 minutes longer then remove from heat. Sweeten to taste, if needed. Strain, cool slightly and serve.

You may refrigerate before serving.

* Please consult your herbal supplier for health warnings regarding licorice root. It is not for prolonged use. If for any reason you can't use licorice root, substitute it in this recipe with 1 tsp fennel seeds.

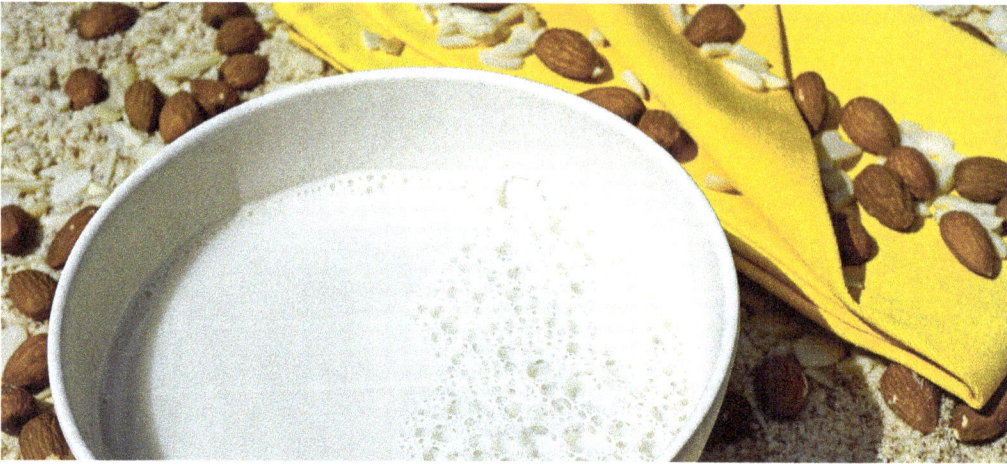

# Upset Stomach Milk 1

1 tsp fennel seed
1/2 tsp dried ginger root
2 cups milk

Mix dried herbs and milk in a small saucepan. You may also place herbs in a tea ball so you don't have to strain them later. Heat on medium/low heat until steaming. Heat 5 minutes longer then remove from heat. Sweeten to taste. Strain, cool slightly and serve.

You may refrigerate before serving.

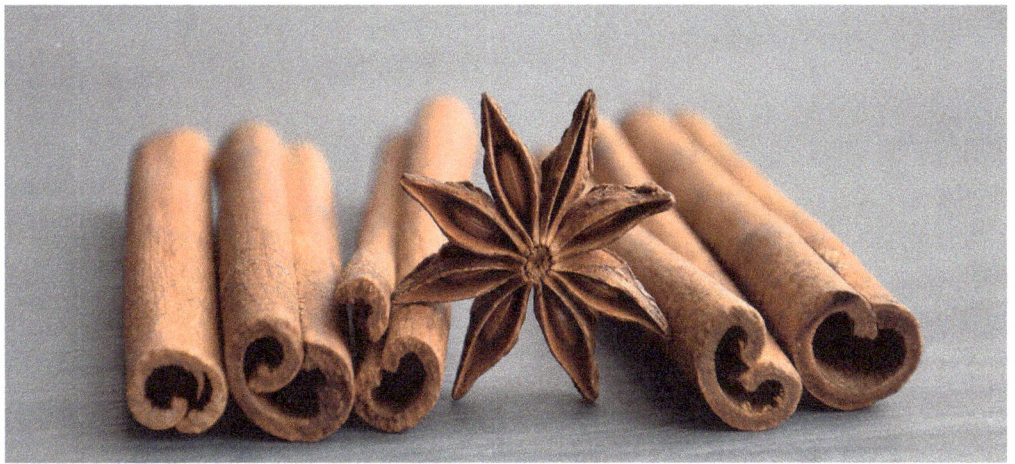

# Upset Stomach Milk 2

1/4 stick cinnamon
2 cups milk


Place cinnamon and milk in a small saucepan. Heat on medium/low heat until steaming. Heat 3 minutes longer then remove from heat. Remove cinnamon. Sweeten to taste. Cool slightly and serve.

You may refrigerate before serving.

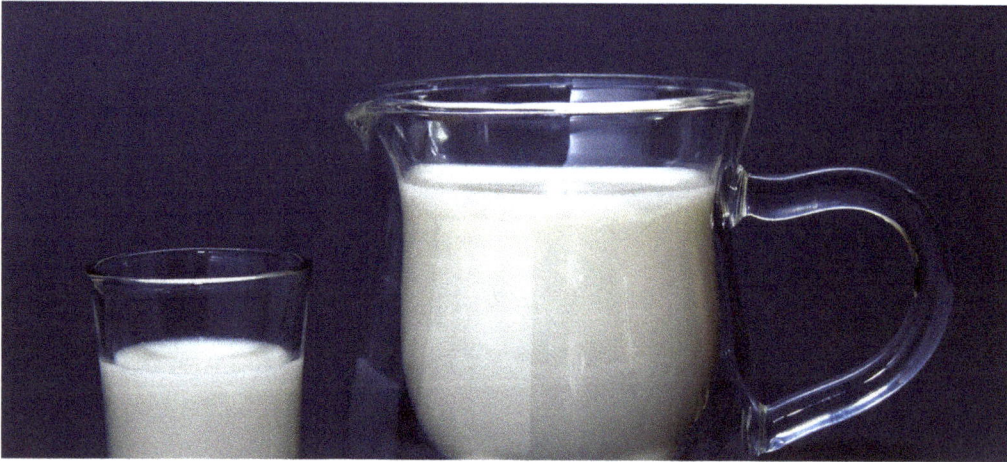

# After Dinner Milk

2 tsp anise seeds
2 cups milk

Mix dried herbs and milk in a small saucepan. You may also place herbs in a tea ball so you don't have to strain them later. Heat on medium/low heat until steaming. Heat 3 minutes longer then remove from heat. Sweeten to taste. Strain, cool slightly and serve.

You may refrigerate before serving.

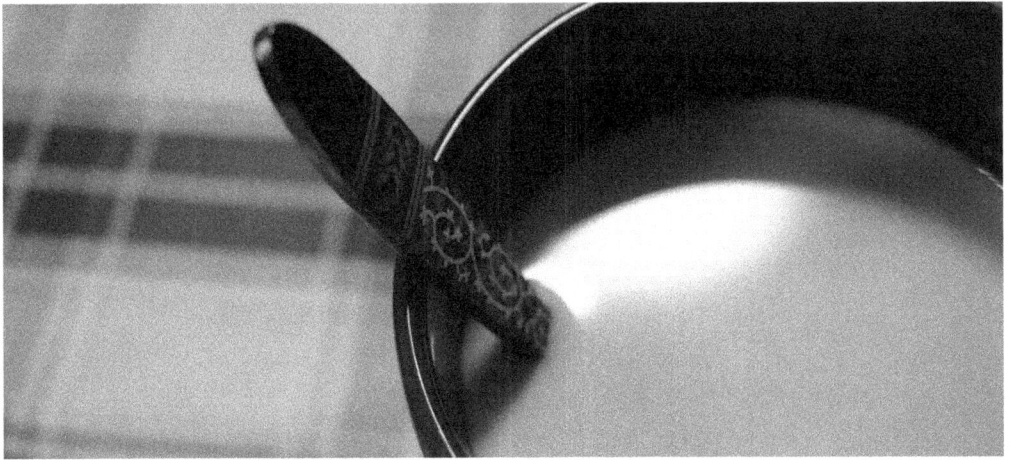

# Bedtime Milk

1/2 tsp dried lavender flowers
  or
1 tsp dried chamomile flowers
2 cups milk


Mix dried herbs and milk in a small saucepan. You may also place herbs in a tea ball so you don't have to strain them later. Heat on medium/low heat until steaming. Heat 3 minutes longer then remove from heat. Sweeten to taste. Strain, cool slightly and serve.

You may refrigerate before serving.

# Cocoas

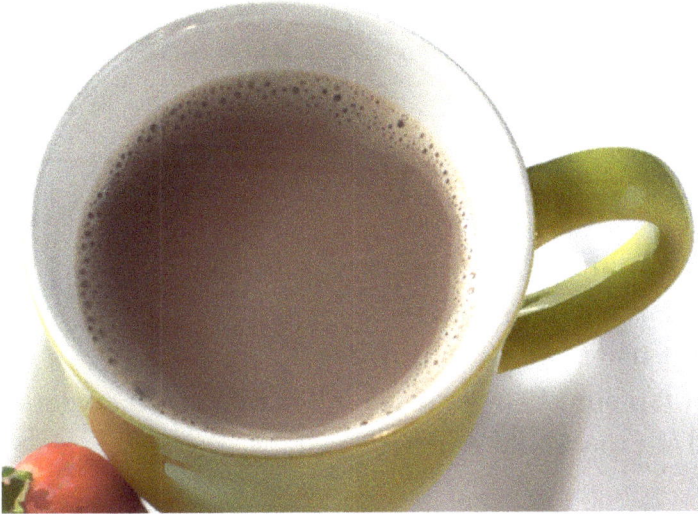

These cocoas are a great way to warm up after a cold day outside. For a dairy-free option you can use almond milk, coconut milk, hemp milk, soy milk, rice milk, oat milk or water.

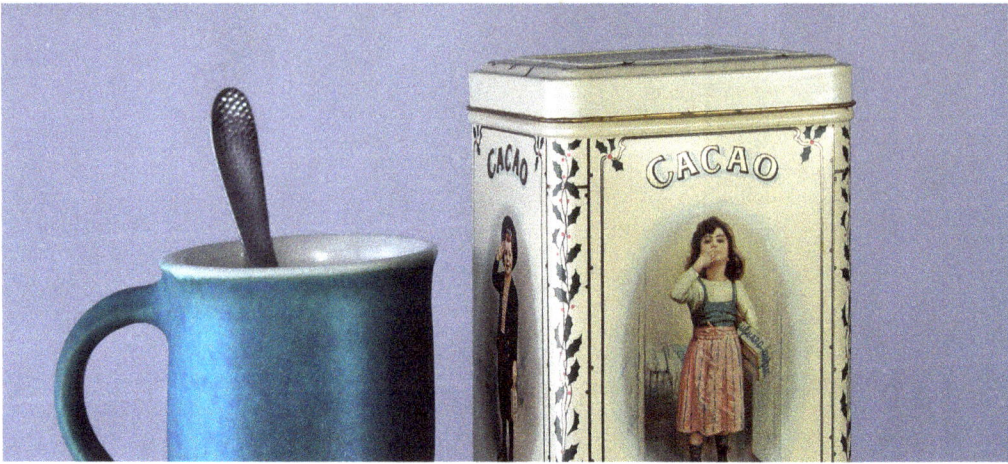

# Cocoa

1 cup milk (or non-dairy option)
4 tsp cocoa powder
~ I use raw cacao powder
4 tsp sugar (or equivalent of preferred sweetener)
1/4 tsp vanilla extract

Combine sugar and cocoa in small bowl. In a saucepan, heat milk over medium/low heat. When steaming, slowly whisk in cocoa and sugar mixture. Add herbs or spices from facing page, if desired, and stir. Reduce heat to low and cover. Stir occasionally. Remove from heat after 10 minutes. Add vanilla. Strain if you used herbs, and serve.

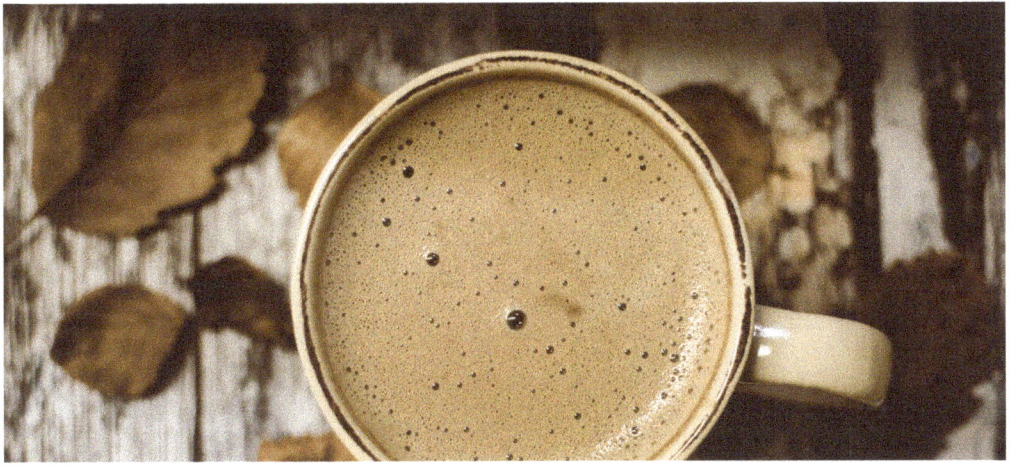

## Spearmint Cocoa
1/2 tsp dried spearmint leaves

## Ginger Cocoa
1/4 tsp dried ginger root

## Lavender Cocoa
1/4 tsp dried lavender flowers

## Hot and Spicy Cocoa
1/8 tsp cinnamon
Dash of cayenne

# Smoothies

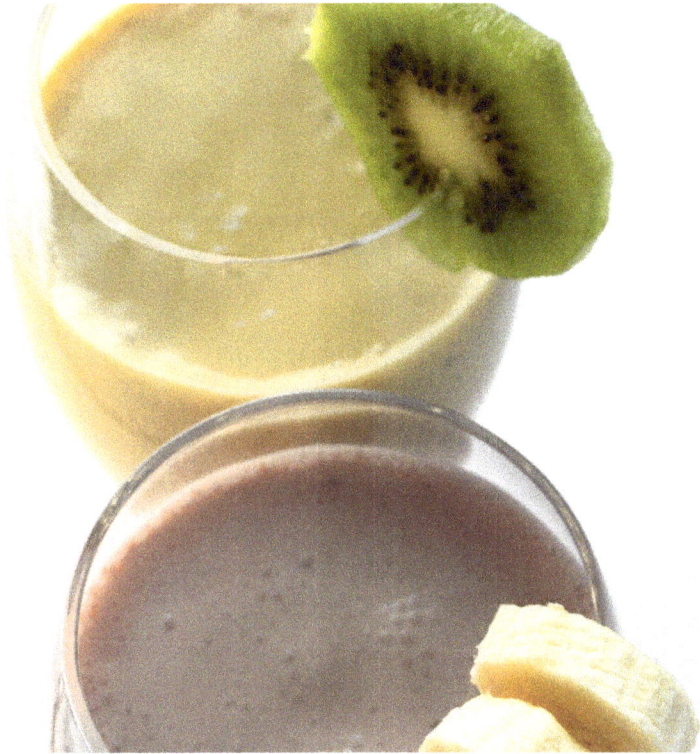

All of the following smoothie recipes are non-dairy, using a hemp milk base. You may use dairy milk or any other non-dairy alternative that you prefer. To add probiotic benefits to the following recipes, add 1 cup of yogurt, kefir or a probiotic supplement and blend.

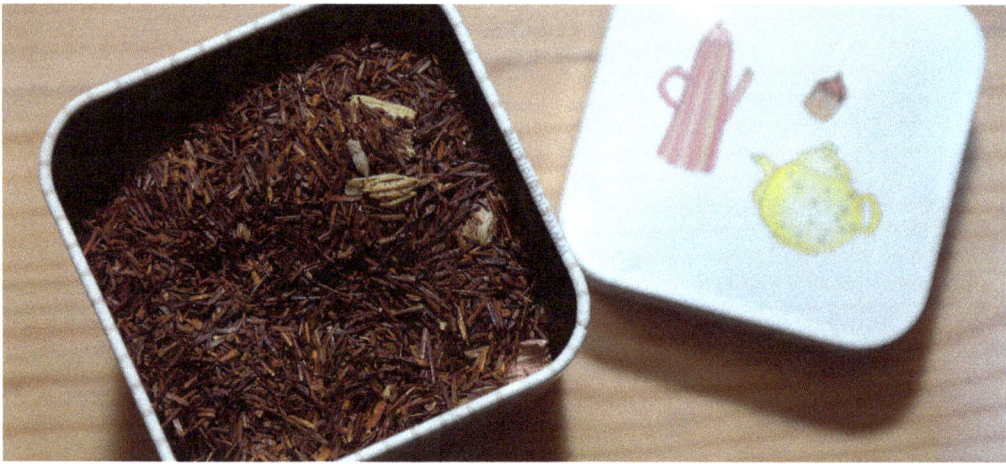

# Chai Smoothie

**Base**
3 Tbsp raw shelled hemp seeds
2 cups water
~ You may use any other dairy or non-dairy milk as
        a base instead

1/4 tsp rooibos tea
1/8 tsp ground cinnamon
1/8 tsp ground ginger
1/8 tsp ground nutmeg
1 Tbsp. sugar, or other sweetener to taste
1 cup ice (optional)

Place all ingredients in a blender. Blend until smooth.
Sweeten to taste.

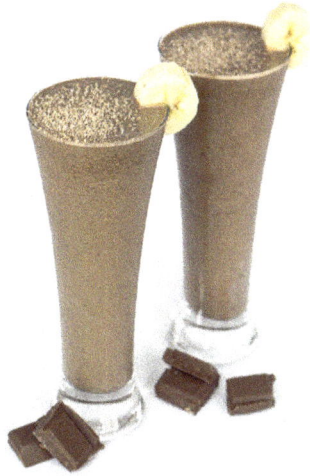

# Chocolate Chai Smoothie

Add 1 tsp Chocolate Syrup (page 94)

# Vanilla Chai Smoothie

Add 1 tsp Vanilla Syrup (page 96)

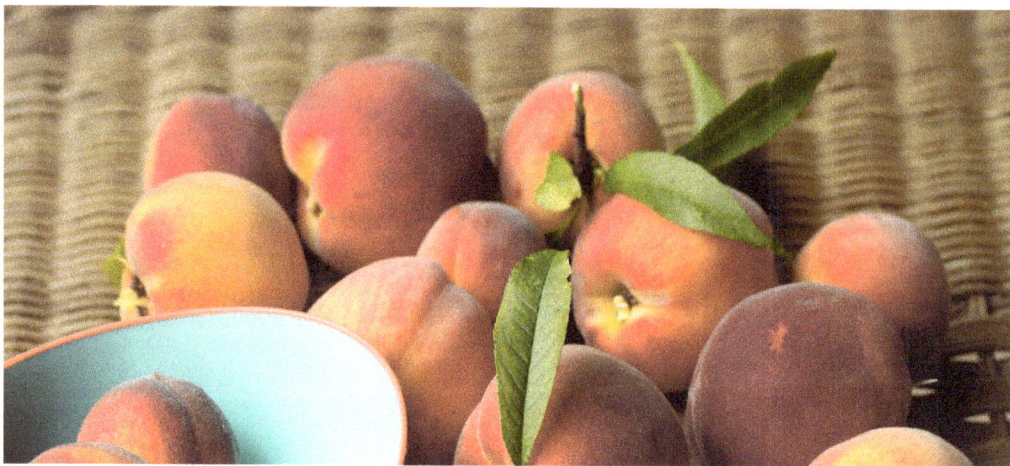

# Upset Stomach Smoothie

**Base**
3 Tbsp raw shelled hemp seeds
2 cups water
~ You may use any other dairy or non-dairy milk as
    a base instead

1/2 cup peaches, fresh or frozen
1/4 tsp dried ginger root
    ~or use 1 tsp Ginger Syrup (page 91)
1 cup ice (optional)

Place all ingredients in a blender. Blend until smooth.

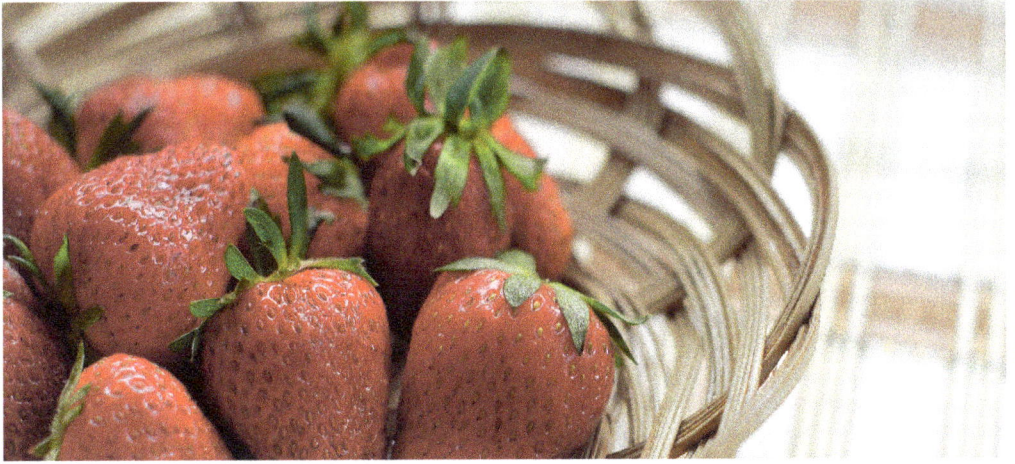

# Antiviral Smoothie

**Base**

3 Tbsp raw shelled hemp seeds

2 cups water

~ You may use any other dairy or non-dairy milk as
a base instead


1/4 tsp dried spearmint

1/2 tsp dried elderberries

1/8 tsp vanilla

1/2 cup fresh or frozen strawberries

1 cup ice (optional)


Place all ingredients in a blender. Blend until smooth.

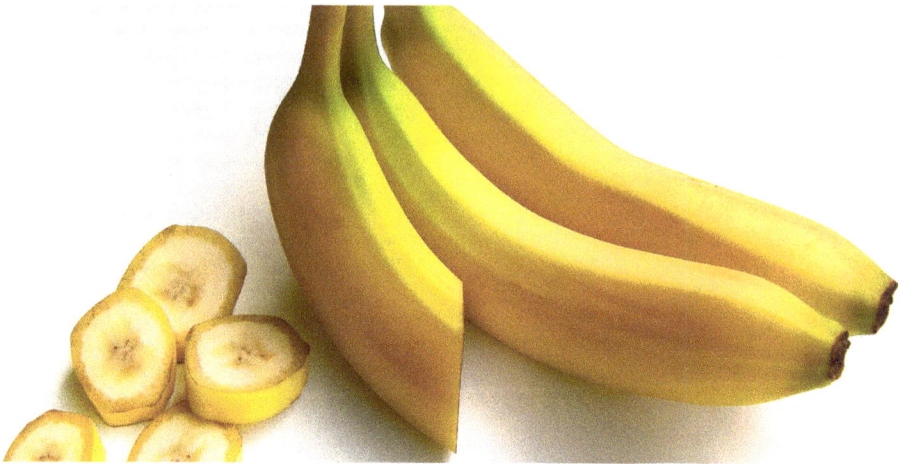

# Cinnamon Burst Smoothie

**Base**

3 Tbsp raw shelled hemp seeds

2 cups water

~ You may use any other dairy or non-dairy milk as
a base instead

1 banana

3 inch piece of cinnamon stick

1/4 tsp nutmeg

1 cup ice

1/3 cup cashews (optional)

Place all ingredients in a blender. Blend until smooth.

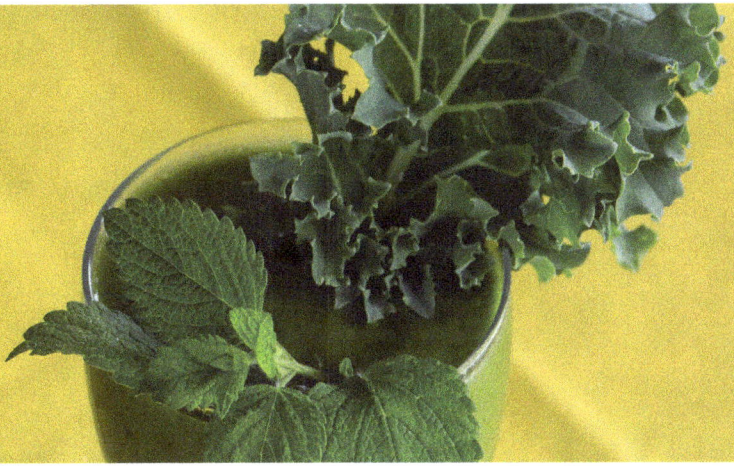

# Morning Rush Smoothie

**Base**

1 Tbsp raw shelled hemp seeds

2 cups water

~ You may use any other dairy or non-dairy milk as
   a base instead

1 peeled orange

1/2 cucumber

handful of kale

1/4 tsp ginger

1/2 tsp rose hips

1 cup ice

Place all ingredients in a blender. Blend until smooth.

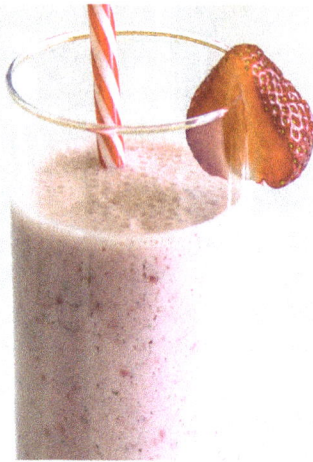

# Clear Skin Refresher Smoothie

**Base**

3 Tbsp raw shelled hemp seeds

2 cups water

~ You may use any other dairy or non-dairy milk as
    a base instead

1 whole apple, peeled if desired

1/2 cucumber, peeled if desired

1/2 tsp dried dandelion root

1/2 cup fresh or frozen strawberries

1 cup ice (optional)

Place all ingredients in a blender. Blend until smooth.

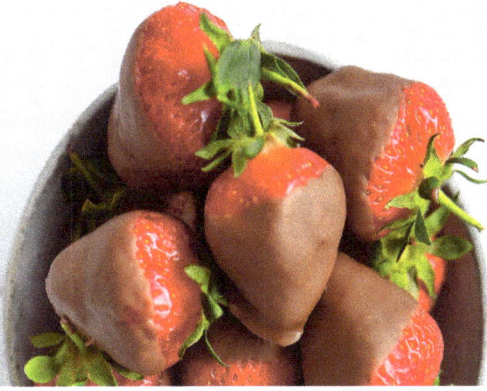

# Chocolate Covered Strawberry Smoothie

**Base**

3 Tbsp raw shelled hemp seeds

2 cups water

~ You may use any other dairy or non-dairy milk as
a base instead

1/4 cup coconut

~ fresh coconut blends best but you can use dried

2 Tbsp raw cacao powder

1/2 ripe avocado

1 1/2 cups fresh or frozen strawberries

1 Tbsp rose hips

1 cup ice (optional)

Sweeten to taste if desired

Place all ingredients in a blender. Blend until smooth.

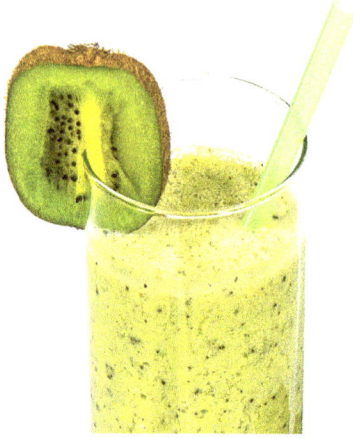

# Banana Kiwi Smoothie

**Base**

3 Tbsp raw shelled hemp seeds

2 cups water

~ You may use any other dairy or non-dairy milk as
    a base instead


1/4 tsp oatstraw

1/4 tsp alfalfa

1/4 tsp nettles

1 peeled kiwi

1/2 banana

1 cup ice


Place all ingredients in a blender. Blend until smooth.

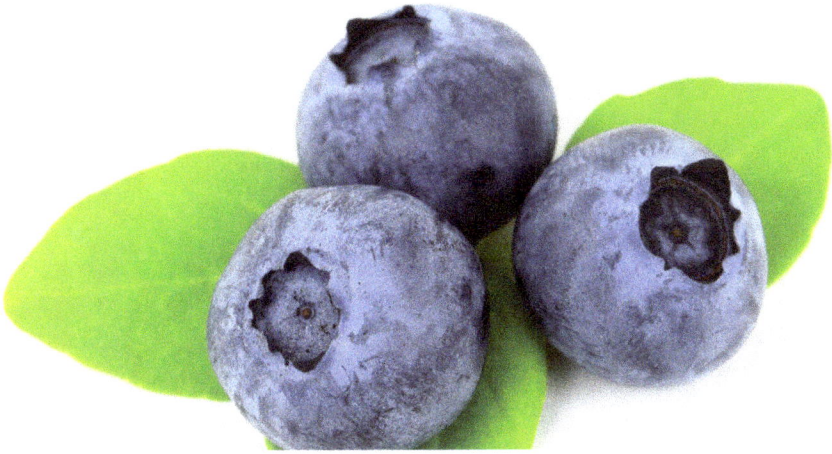

# Blueberry Blast Smoothie

**Base**

3 Tbsp raw shelled hemp seeds

2 cups water

~ You may use any other dairy or non-dairy milk as
   a base instead

1 cup fresh or frozen blueberries

1 whole peeled banana

3 Tbsp raw cacao powder

1 cup ice

Place all ingredients in a blender. Blend until smooth.

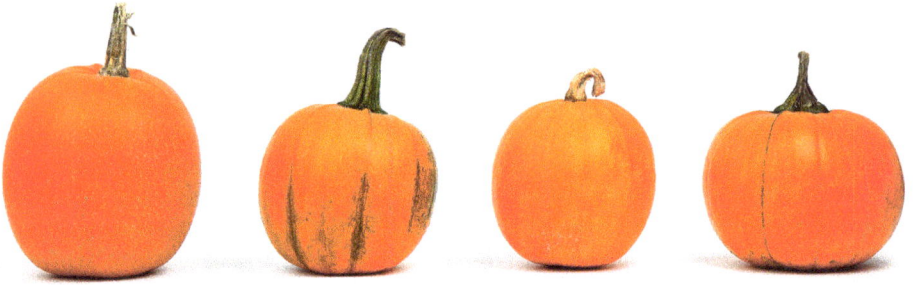

# Pumpkin Smoothie

**Base**

3 Tbsp raw shelled hemp seeds

2 cups water

~ You may use any other dairy or non-dairy milk as
  a base instead


1 cup pureed pumpkin

1/2 tsp ground cinnamon

1/2 tsp ground nutmeg

1/2 ripe banana

1 cup ice (optional)


Place all ingredients in a blender. Blend until smooth.

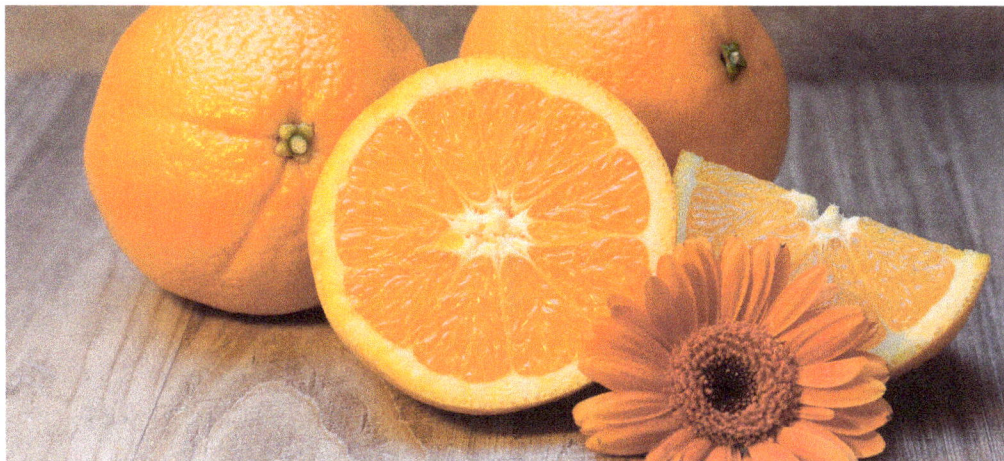

# Power Up Vitamin C Smoothie

**Base**

2 Tbsp raw shelled hemp seeds

1 cup water

~ You may use any other non-dairy milk as
    a base instead

\*\* Do not use dairy due to the lemon juice


2 large peeled oranges

2 tsp rose hips

1 Tbsp lemon juice

1/4 cup pomegranate or cranberry juice

1/2 cup ice


Place all ingredients in a blender. Blend until smooth.

# Iced Teas

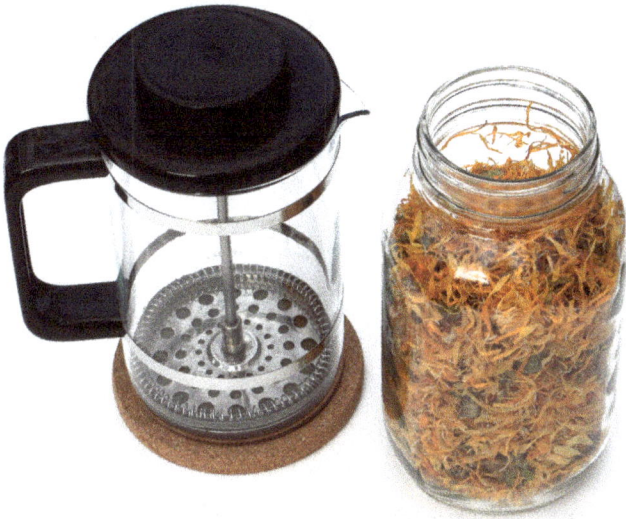

The following iced teas can be easily made in a French press, like the one pictured above. However, you can also use a saucepan and strainer. You can also make a sun tea by placing the herbs in a covered pitcher of water to brew in the summer sun.

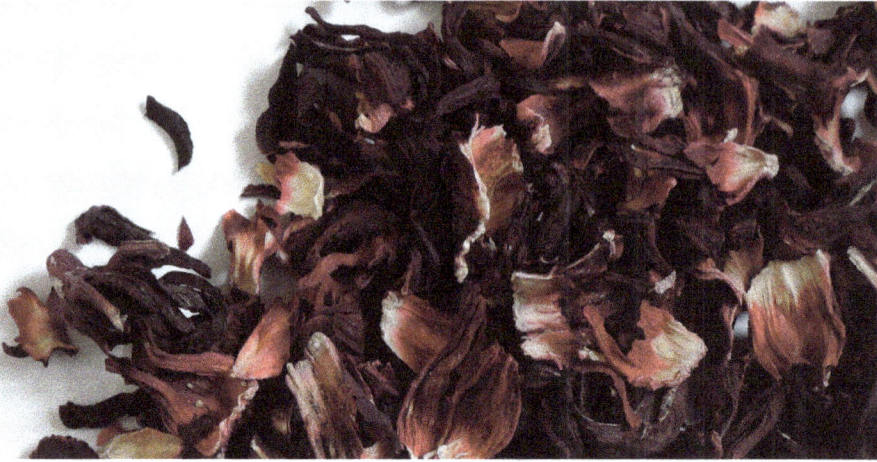

# Croc-Aid

4 Tbsp dried hibiscus
1/2 cup sugar (or other sweetener to taste)
2 limes - quartered (if desired)

Yield: 2 quarts

Place hibiscus and sweetener into a French press; or you can use a small saucepan. Pour approximately 2 cups of hot water over the tea and stir until the sweetener is dissolved. Let sit for at least 5 minutes. Strain liquid into two-quart pitcher that is filled with ice cubes. Fill the balance with water. Add limes. Mix well.

This is a great replacement for less nutritious and artificially colored drinks. Kids love it because it's bright red. This tea mixes well with any other herbs you would like to add. It also makes great popsicles. Pour in molds and add berries.

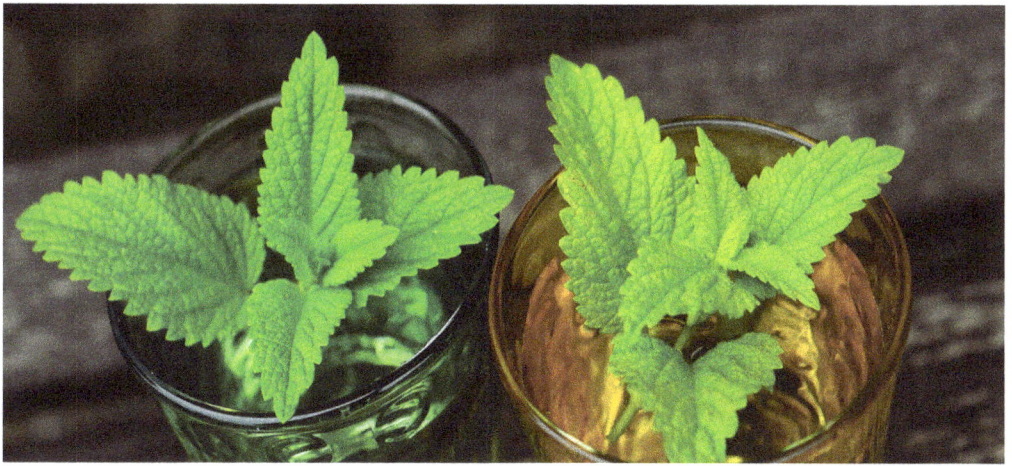

# Rose Hips Iced Tea

1/4 cup dried lemon balm
1/3 cup dried seedless rose hips
1/4 cup lemon juice
1/3 cup sugar (or other sweetener to taste)

Yield: 2 quarts

Place lemon balm, rose hips and sweetener into a
French press; or you can use a small saucepan. Pour
approximately 2 cups of hot water over the tea and stir
until the sweetener is dissolved. Let sit for 20 minutes.
Strain liquid into two-quart pitcher that is filled with ice
cubes. Add lemon juice and fill the balance with water.
Mix well.

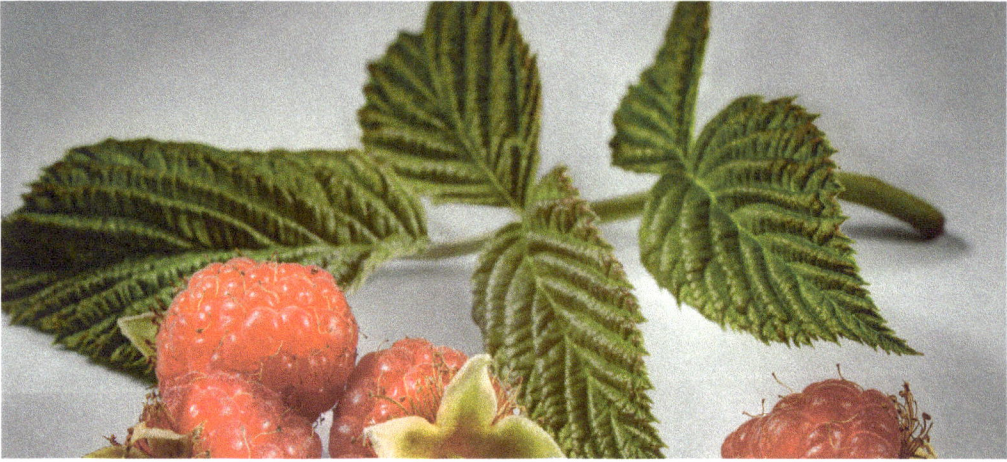

# Red Raspberry Leaf Iced Tea

6 Tbsp red raspberry leaf
1 Tbsp spearmint leaf (optional)
1/8 cup sugar (or other sweetener to taste)

Yield: 2 quarts

Place red raspberry leaf, spearmint, if desired, and sweetener into a French press; or you can use a small saucepan. Pour approximately 2 cups of hot water over the tea and stir until the sweetener is dissolved. Let sit for 20 minutes. Strain liquid into two-quart pitcher that is filled with ice cubes. Fill the balance with water. Mix well.

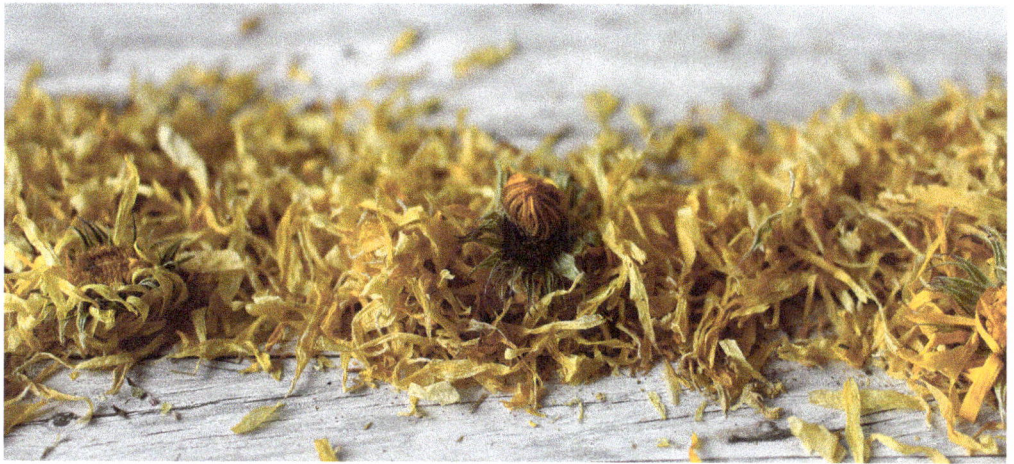

# Calendula & Hibiscus Iced Tea

3 Tbsp dried calendula flowers
1 Tbsp dried hibiscus
1/3 cup sugar (or other sweetener to taste)

Yield: 2 quarts

Place calendula, hibiscus, and sweetener into a
French press; or you can use a small saucepan. Pour
approximately 2 cups of hot water over the tea and stir
until the sweetener is dissolved. Let sit for 20 minutes.
Strain liquid into two-quart pitcher that is filled with ice
cubes. Fill the balance with water. Mix well.

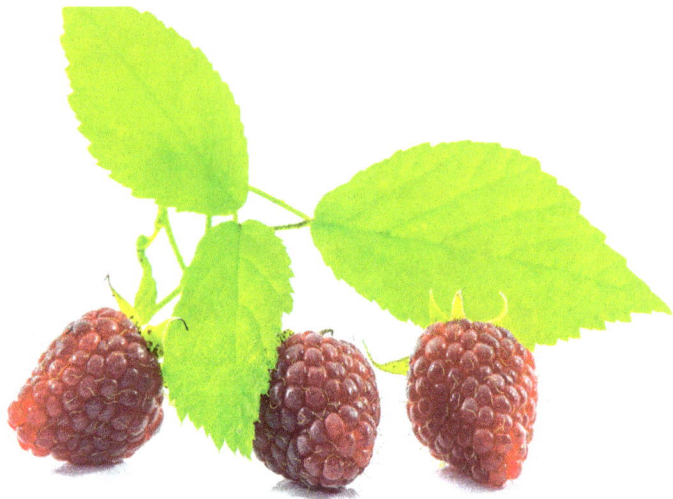

# Ginger & Red Raspberry Leaf Iced Tea

1 Tbsp dried ginger root
1/3 cup dried red raspberry leaf
1/3 cup sugar (or other sweetener to taste)

Yield: 2 quarts

Place ginger, red raspberry leaf, and sweetener into a French press; or you can use a small saucepan. Pour approximately 2 cups of hot water over the tea and stir until the sweetener is dissolved. Let sit for 20 minutes. Strain liquid into two-quart pitcher that is filled with ice cubes. Fill the balance with water. Mix well.

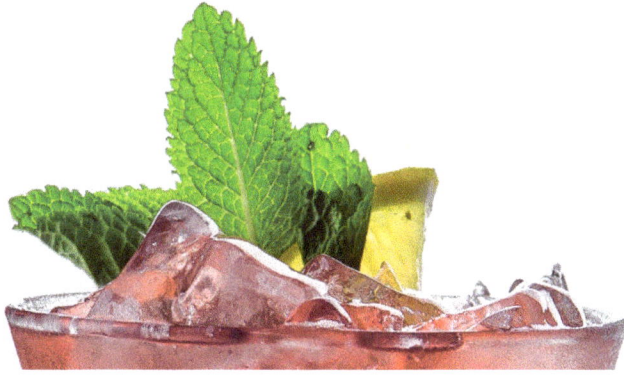

# Elderberry Iced Tea

1/4 cup dried elderberries
3 Tbsp. dried lemon balm
1/3 cup sugar (or other sweetener to taste)

Yield: 2 quarts

Place elderberries, lemon balm, and sweetener into a French press; or you can use a small saucepan. Pour approximately 2 cups of hot water over the tea and stir until the sweetener is dissolved. Let sit for 20 minutes. Strain liquid into two-quart pitcher that is filled with ice cubes. Fill the balance with water. Mix well.

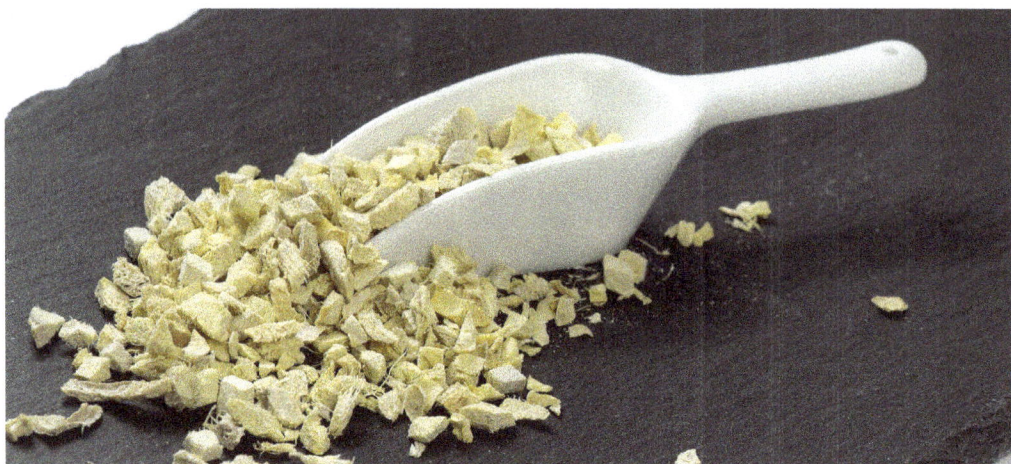

# Ginger Oatstraw Iced Tea

4 tsp dried oatstraw
2 tsp dried ginger root
1/3 cup sugar (or other sweetener to taste)

Yield: 2 quarts

Place oatstraw, ginger and sweetener into a French press; or you can use a small saucepan. Pour approximately 2 cups of hot water over the tea and stir until the sweetener is dissolved. Let sit for 20 minutes. Strain liquid into two-quart pitcher that is filled with ice cubes. Fill the balance with water. Mix well.

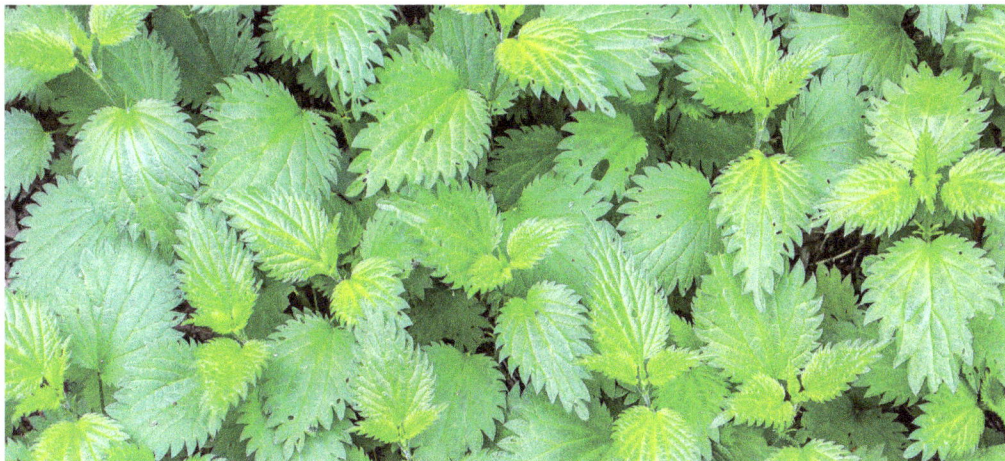

# Nettles and Rose Hips Iced Tea

4 tsp dried nettles
4 tsp dried rose hips
1/2 cup sugar (or other sweetener to taste)

Yield: 2 quarts

Place nettles, rose hips and sweetener into a French press;
or you can use a small saucepan. Pour approximately 2
cups of hot water over the tea and stir until the sweetener
is dissolved. Let sit for 10 minutes. Strain liquid into a two-
quart pitcher that is filled with ice cubes. Fill the balance
with water. Mix well.

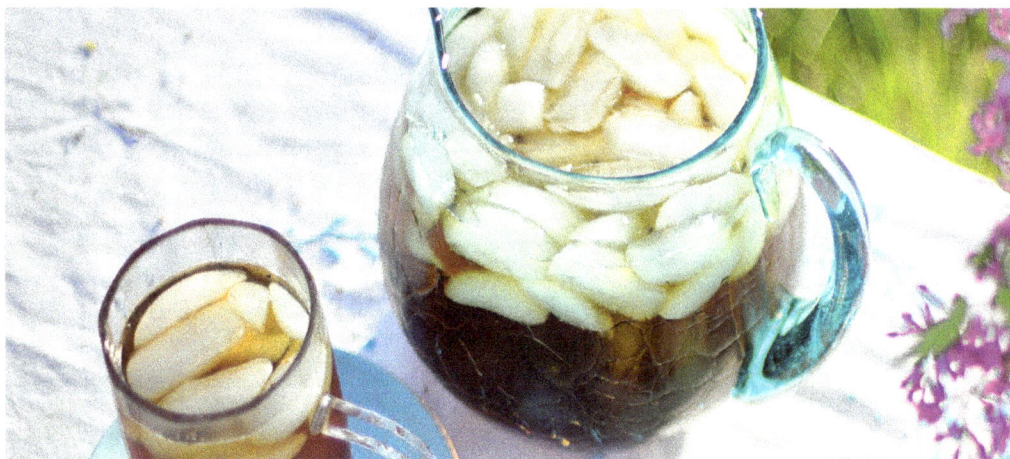

# Iced Chai

4 tsp rooibos tea
6 whole cloves
1 cinnamon stick - broken up
1/2 tsp dried ginger root
6 whole cardamom pods - broken up
1/2 tsp ground nutmeg
1/2 cup brown sugar
1 cup milk (dairy or non-dairy, if desired)

Yield: 2 quarts

Place tea, herbs, spices and sweetener into a French press; or you can use a small saucepan. Pour approximately 2 cups of hot water over the tea and stir until the sweetener is dissolved. Let sit for 10 minutes. Strain liquid into a two-quart pitcher that is filled with ice cubes. Add milk, if desired, and fill the balance with water. Mix well.

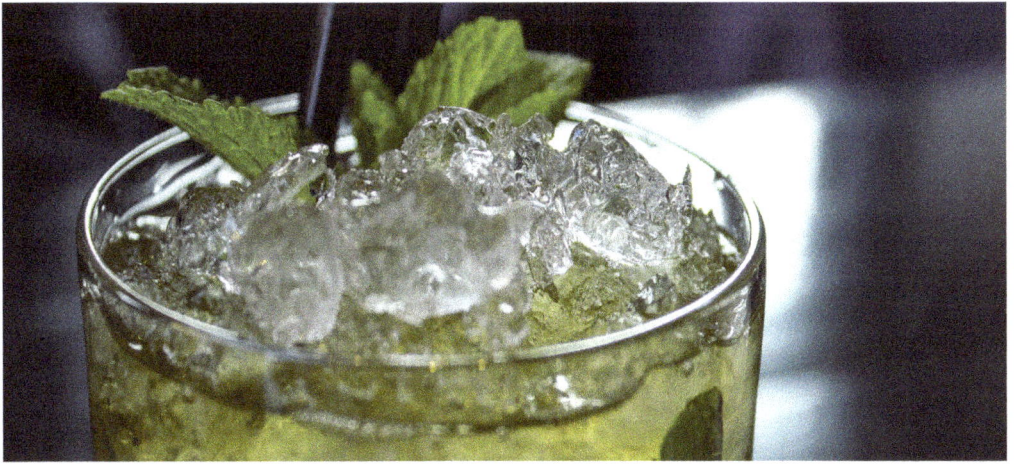

# After Dinner Iced Tea

4 tsp dried lemon balm
4 tsp dried red raspberry leaf
1/4 cup sugar (or other sweetener to taste)

Yield: 2 quarts

Place lemon balm, red raspberry leaf and sweetener into a French press; or you can use a small saucepan. Pour approximately 2 cups of hot water over the tea and stir until the sweetener is dissolved. Let sit for 10 minutes. Strain liquid into two-quart pitcher that is filled with ice cubes. Fill the balance with water. Mix well.

# Lemonades

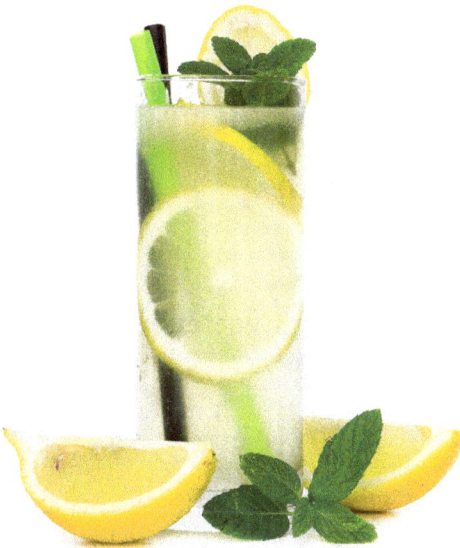

These great tasting lemonades can be enjoyed daily any time of year. Pour into popsicle molds and add fruit for a healthy summer treat.

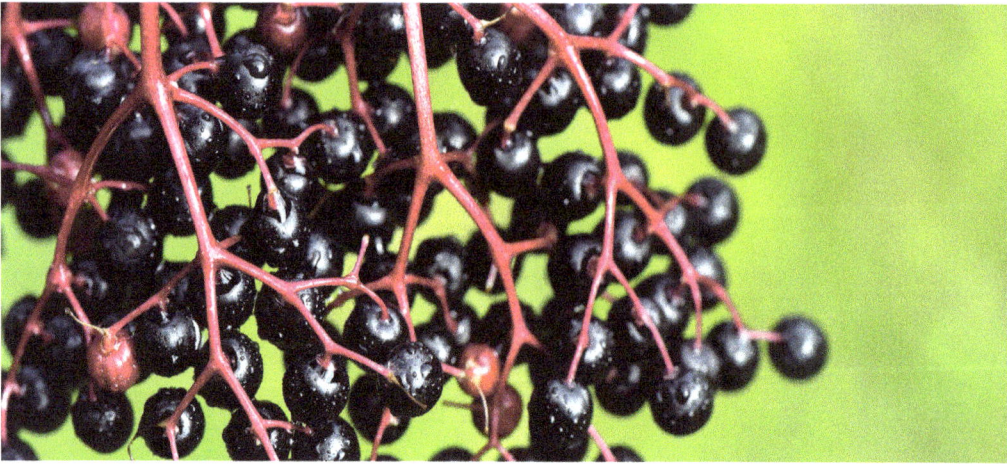

# Elderberry Lemonade

1/3 cup dried elderberries
2 cups boiling water
1/3 cup lemon juice
1/3 cup sugar (or other sweetener to taste)

Yield: 2 quarts

Place elderberries and sugar into a French press; or you can use a small saucepan. Pour 2 cups of hot water over the elderberries and stir until the sweetener is dissolved. Let sit for 20 minutes. Strain liquid into a two-quart pitcher that is filled with ice cubes. Add lemon juice and fill the balance with water. Mix well.

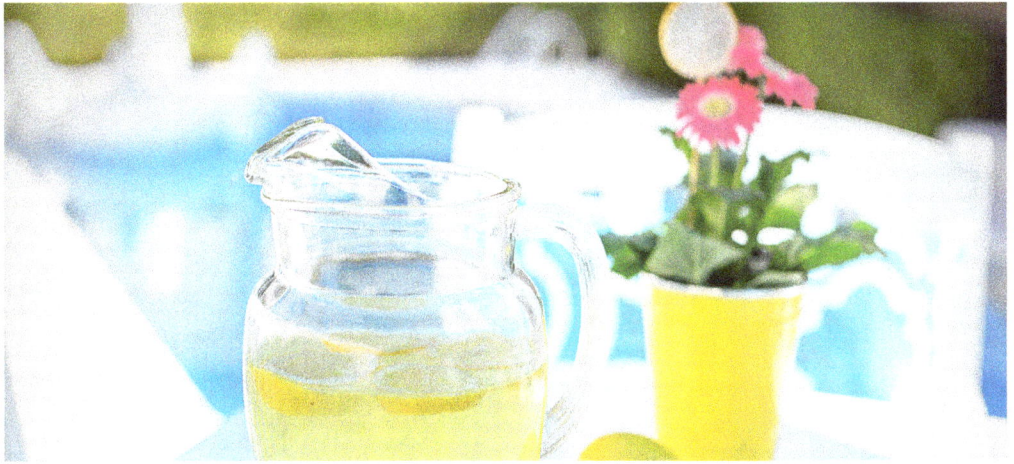

# Red Raspberry Leaf Lemonade

1/3 cup dried red raspberry leaf
2 cups boiling water
1/2 cup lemon juice
1/3 cup sugar (or other sweetener to taste)

Yield: 2 quarts

Place red raspberry leaf and sugar into a French press; or you can use a small saucepan. Pour 2 cups of hot water over the red raspberry leaf and stir until the sweetener is dissolved. Let sit for 15 minutes. Strain liquid into a two-quart pitcher that is filled with ice cubes. Add lemon juice and fill the balance with water. Mix well.

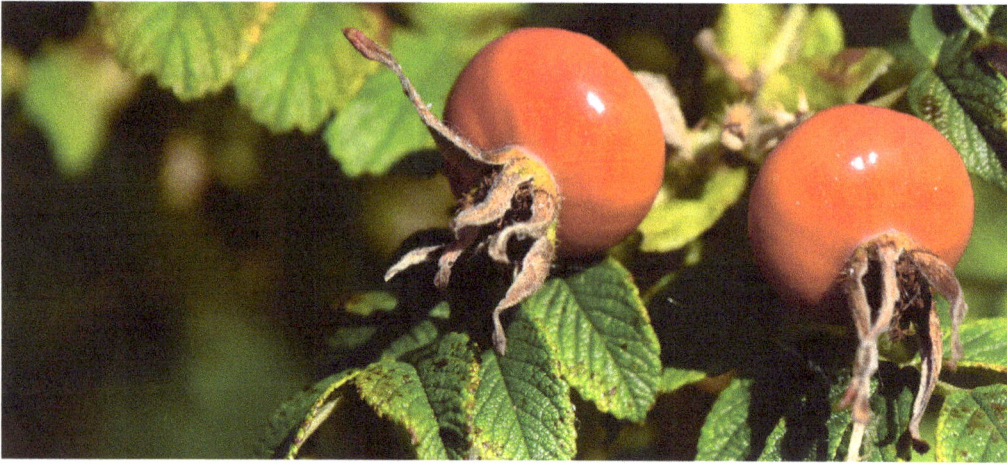

# Rose Hips Lemonade

1/4 cup dried rose hips
2 cups boiling water
1/2 cup lemon juice
1/2 cup sugar (or other sweetener to taste)

Yield: 2 quarts

Place rose hips and sugar into a French press; or you can use a small saucepan. Pour 2 cups of hot water over the rose hips and stir until the sweetener is dissolved. Let sit for 20 minutes. Strain liquid into a two-quart pitcher that is filled with ice cubes. Add lemon juice and fill the balance with water. Mix well.

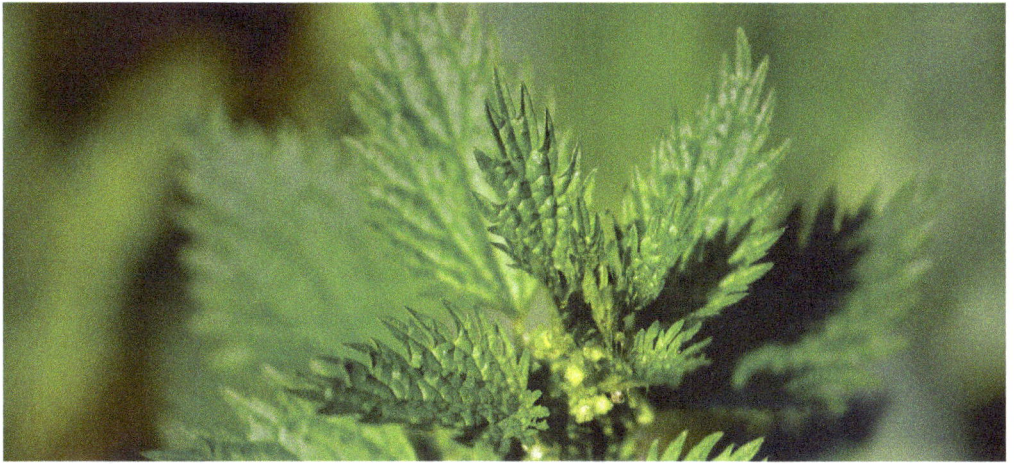

# Nettles Lemonade

4 Tbsp dried nettles
2 cups boiling water
1/2 cup lemon juice
1/2 cup sugar (or other sweetener to taste)

Yield: 2 quarts

Place nettles and sugar into a French press; or you can use a small saucepan. Pour 2 cups of hot water over the nettles and stir until the sweetener is dissolved. Let sit for 20 minutes. Strain liquid into a two-quart pitcher that is filled with ice cubes. Add lemon juice and fill the balance with water. Mix well.

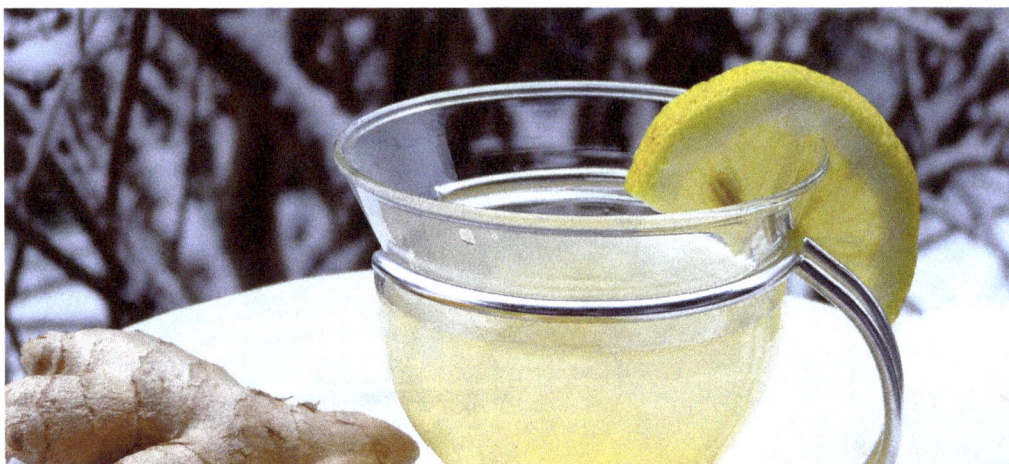

# Ginger Lemonade

1 Tbsp dried ginger root
2 cups boiling water
1/2 cup lemon juice
1/2 cup sugar (or other sweetener to taste)

Yield: 2 quarts

Place ginger and sugar into a French press; or you can use a small saucepan. Pour 2 cups of hot water over the ginger and stir until the sweetener is dissolved. Let sit for 15 minutes. Strain liquid into a two-quart pitcher that is filled with ice cubes. Add lemon juice and fill the balance with water. Mix well.

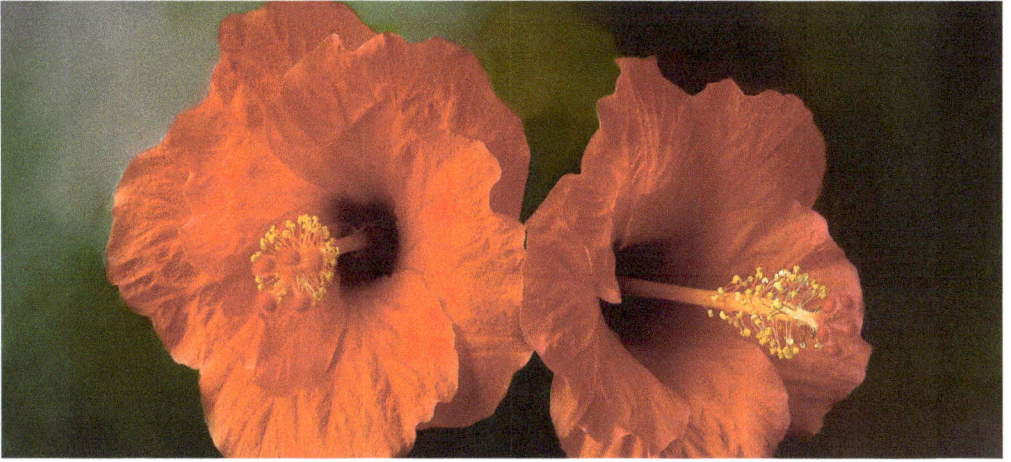

# Pink Lemonade

4 Tbsp dried hibiscus
2 cups boiling water
1/2 cup lemon juice
1/2 cup sugar (or other sweetener to taste)

Yield: 2 quarts

Place hibiscus and sugar into a French press; or you can use a small saucepan. Pour 2 cups of hot water over the hibiscus and stir until the sweetener is dissolved. Let sit for 20 minutes. Strain liquid into a two-quart pitcher that is filled with ice cubes. Add lemon juice and fill the balance with water. Mix well.

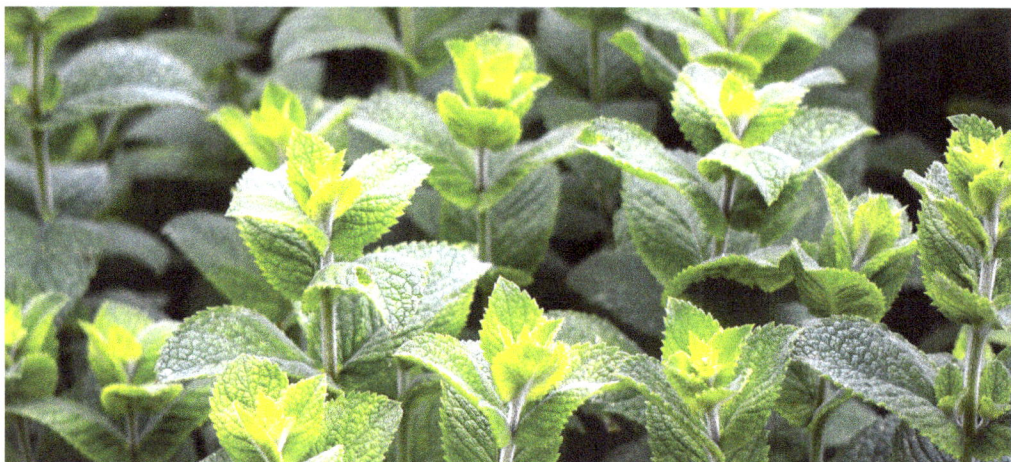

# Mint Lemonade

4 tsp dried spearmint leaves
2 cups boiling water
1/2 cup lemon juice
1/2 cup sugar (or other sweetener to taste)

Yield: 2 quarts

Place spearmint and sugar into a French press; or you can use a small saucepan. Pour 2 cups of hot water over the spearmint and stir until the sweetener is dissolved. Let sit for 20 minutes. Strain liquid into a two-quart pitcher that is filled with ice cubes. Add lemon juice and fill the balance with water. Mix well.

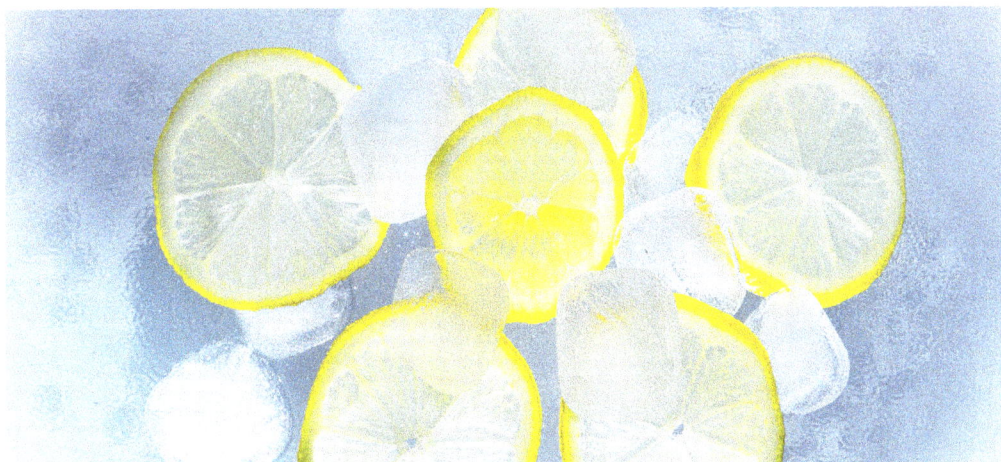

# Rosemary Lemonade

2 tsp dried or fresh rosemary
2 cups boiling water
1/2 cup lemon juice
1/2 cup sugar (or other sweetener to taste)

Yield: 2 quarts

Place rosemary and sugar into a French press; or you can use a small saucepan. Pour 2 cups of hot water over the rosemary and stir until the sweetener is dissolved. Let sit for 10 minutes. Strain liquid into a two-quart pitcher that is filled with ice cubes. Add lemon juice and fill the balance with water. Mix well.

# Syrups

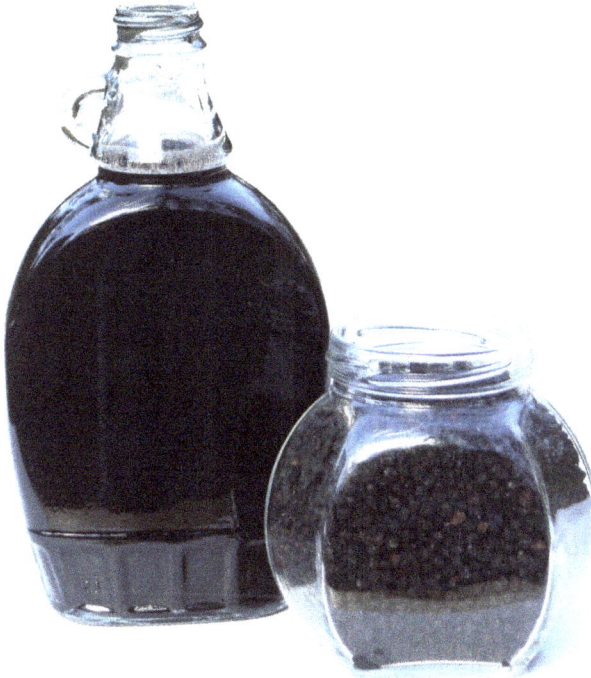

In several of the following recipes, I used sugar due to its ability to create that syrupy consistency when boiled down. Feel free to substitute with raw honey or stevia but keep in mind that the consistency will be much thinner.

For the syrups that use honey as the sweetener, I recommend using local raw honey. Not only does it taste better but it can also help with allergies.

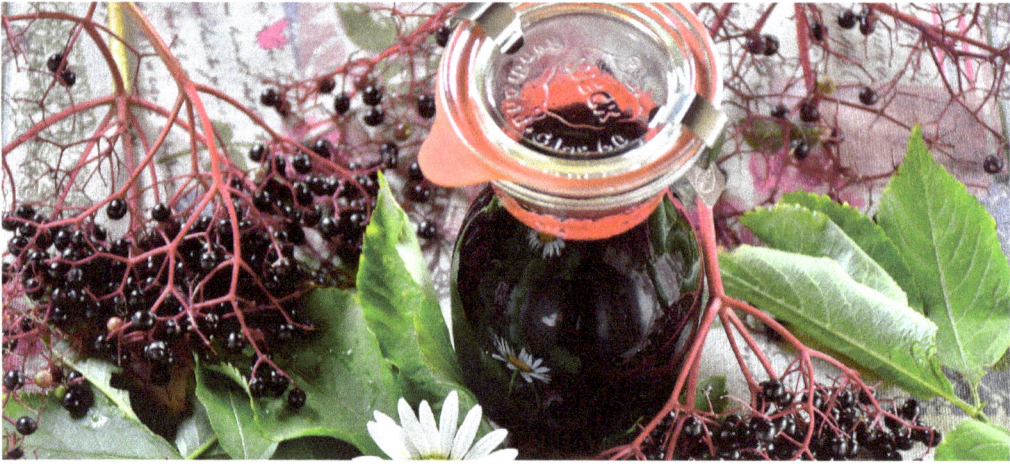

# Elderberry Syrup

3 cups water
1/2 cup dried elderberries
1/2 cinnamon stick
1/2 cup sugar
1/2 cup raw honey

Yield: approx 2 cups

In a medium saucepan, combine everything except honey. Bring to a boil. Reduce heat to a simmer, partially cover and reduce liquid by half. Remove from heat and cool for 15 minutes. Strain liquid into a 2-cup, liquid measuring cup. Add honey and stir until dissolved. Using a kitchen funnel, pour into a serving container. Refrigerate.

Great over yogurt, ice cream, pancakes and waffles! Elderberries are great for boosting your immunity.

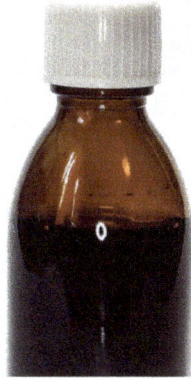

# Expectorant Cough Syrup

3 cups water
2 Tbsp dried marshmallow root
2 Tbsp dried licorice root*
2 Tbsp fennel seed
1/2 cup raw honey

Yield: approx 2 cups

In a medium saucepan, combine ingredients and bring to a boil. Reduce heat to a simmer, partially cover and reduce liquid by half. Remove from heat and cool for 15 minutes. Strain liquid into a 2-cup, liquid measuring cup, or another saucepan. Using a kitchen funnel, pour into a serving container. Refrigerate. Try 1 tsp per hour for relief.

* Please consult your herbal supplier for health warnings regarding licorice root. It is not for prolonged use.

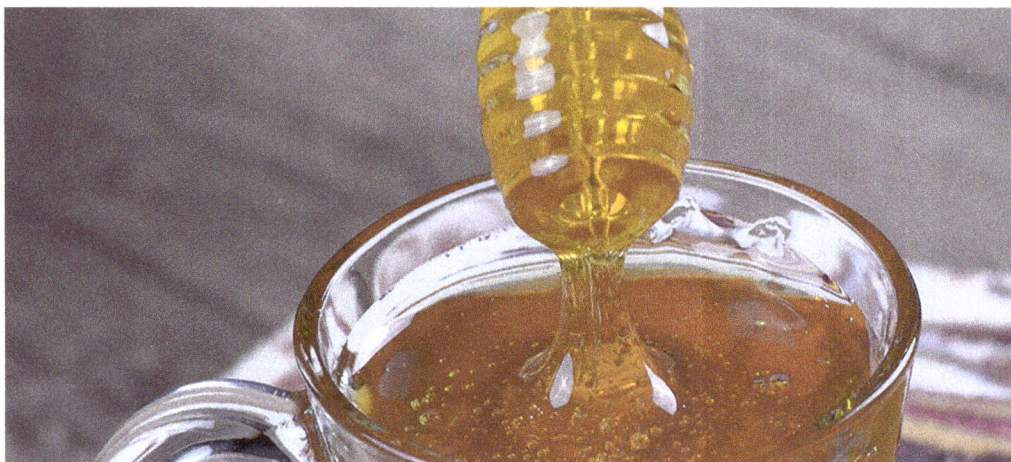

# Suppressant Cough Syrup

3 cups water
2 Tbsp dried wild cherry bark
2 Tbsp anise seed
1 tsp dried ginger root
1/2 cup raw honey
1/2 cup cherry juice

Yield: approx 3 cups

In a medium saucepan, combine all ingredients except for cherry juice and bring to a boil. Reduce heat to a simmer, partially cover and reduce liquid by half. Remove from heat and cool for 15 minutes. Strain liquid into a 4-cup liquid measuring cup, or another saucepan. Add cherry juice. Using a kitchen funnel, pour into a serving container. Refrigerate.

Try 1 tsp per hour for relief. Not for prolonged use!

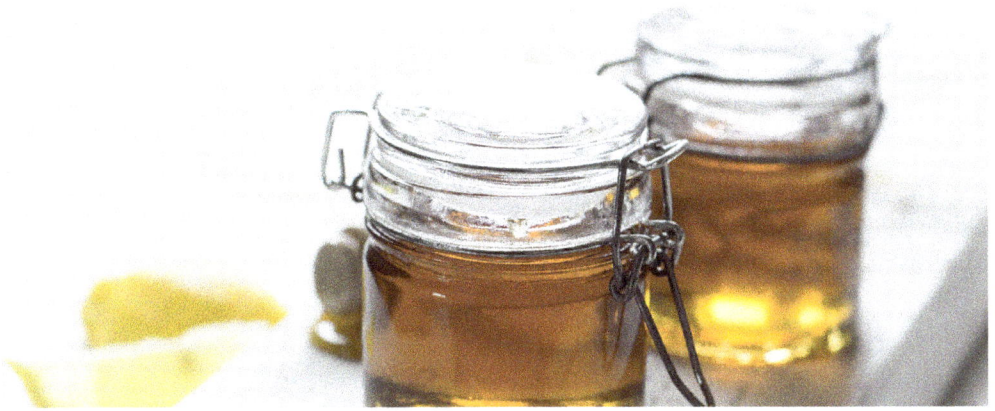

# Ginger Syrup

2 cups water
1 tsp dried ginger root
2 cups sugar

Yield: approx 1 cup

In a medium saucepan, mix together water, sugar and ginger. Bring to a boil while stirring. Reduce heat and simmer until liquid is reduced by half. Remove from heat and let cool on stove for 20 minutes. Strain liquid into a 2-cup, liquid measuring cup, or another saucepan. Using a kitchen funnel, pour into a serving container. Refrigerate.

Taken by itself, 1/2 tsp can relieve nausea and gas. Add to Chamomile tea for headaches, constipation or heartburn.

Try adding this to cold milk!

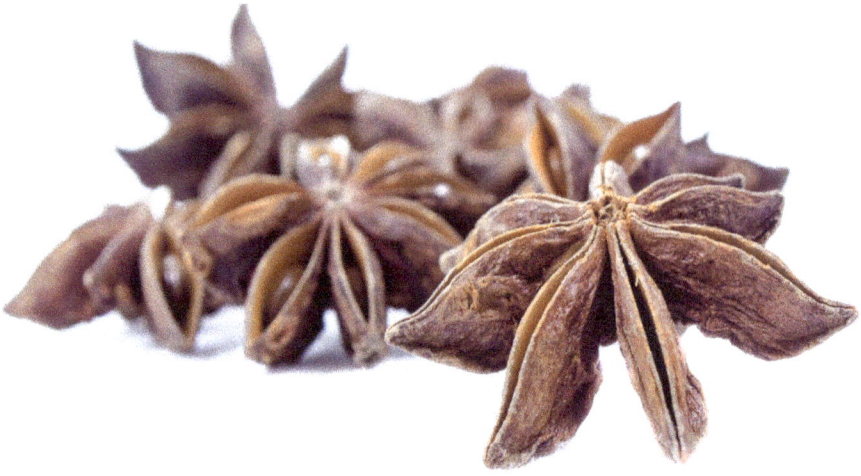

# Stomach Soother Syrup

2 cups water
1 tsp fennel seed
1 tsp anise seed
2 cups sugar

Yield: approx 1 cup

In a medium saucepan, mix together water and sugar. Over high heat, whisk sugar until dissolved. Bring to a boil. Reduce heat and simmer partially covered until liquid is reduced by half. Add fennel and anise and let simmer for 5 more minutes. Remove from heat and let cool 15 minutes. Strain liquid into a 2-cup, liquid measuring cup, or another saucepan. After the syrup is completely cooled, pour into a glass bottle, using a funnel if necessary. Refrigerate.

Taken by itself, 1/2 tsp can relieve nausea and gas. Add to Elderberry tea for cold or flu.

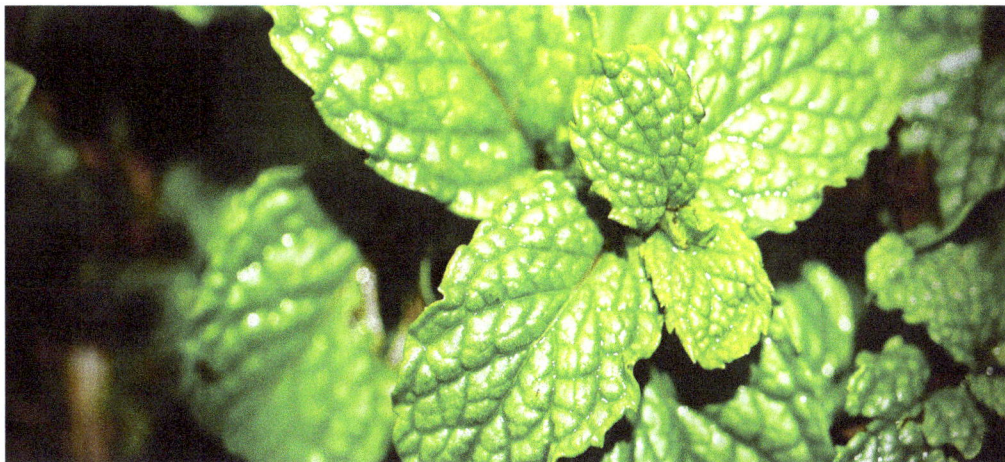

# Spearmint Syrup

2 cups water
1 tsp dried spearmint leaf
2 cups sugar

Yield: approx 1 cup

In a medium saucepan, mix together water, sugar and spearmint. Bring to a boil while stirring. Reduce heat and simmer until liquid is reduced by half. Remove from heat and let cool on stove for 20 minutes. Strain liquid into a 2-cup, liquid measuring cup, or another saucepan. Using a kitchen funnel, pour into a serving container. Refrigerate.

Taken by itself, 1 tsp can relieve nausea and gas.
Add to Lemon Balm tea for gas or stomachache.

Great in cocoa! (see page 47)

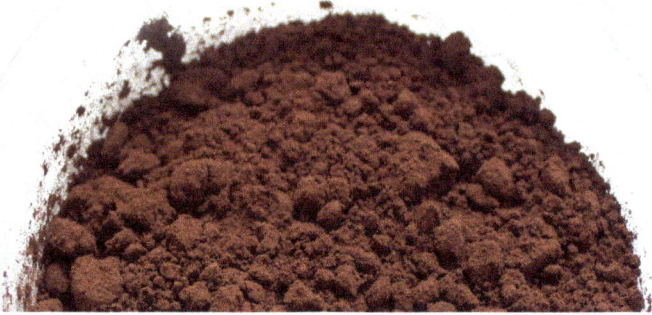

# Chocolate Syrup

1 1/2 cups water
1 1/2 cups non-dutch cocoa powder*
1 tsp vanilla
1 1/2 cups sugar

Yield: approx 2 cups

In a medium saucepan, mix together water and sugar.
Bring to a boil while stirring. Remove from heat and whisk
in cocoa powder 1/2 cup at a time. If too the syrup is too
thin, simmer over low heat until it thickens. Add vanilla.
Cool on stove for 20 minutes. Using a kitchen funnel, pour
into a serving container. Refrigerate.

*Dutch processed cocoa will yield a much thicker result.
If you use it and your syrup is too thick, add 1/2 cup water.

Add this syrup to the chai recipe on page 24 to make your
own chocolate chai!

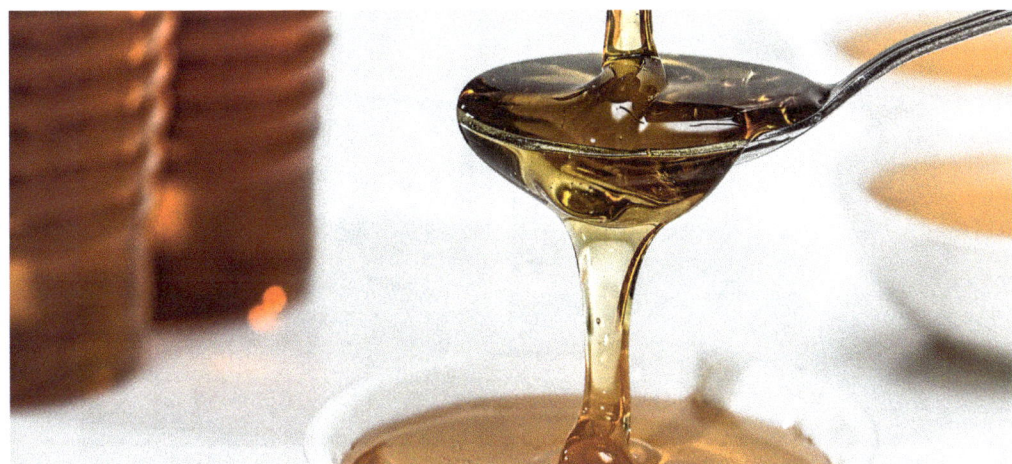

# Simple Syrup

3 cups water
3 cups sugar

Yield: approx 2 cups

In a medium saucepan, mix together water and sugar.
Bring to a boil while stirring. Reduce heat and simmer
until liquid is reduced by half. Remove from heat and cool
on stove for 20 minutes. Using a kitchen funnel, pour into
a serving container. Refrigerate.

This syrup is great to have on hand to sweeten cold
beverages such as iced teas, lemonades, and even iced
coffee.

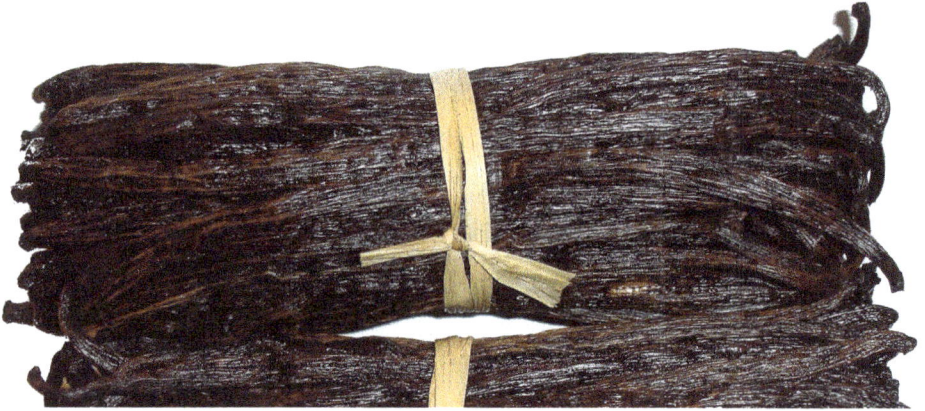

# Vanilla Syrup

1 1/2 cups water
2 tsp vanilla
1 1/2 cups sugar

Yield: approx 1 cup

In a medium saucepan, mix together water and sugar. Bring to a boil while stirring. Reduce heat and simmer until liquid is reduced by half. Remove from heat and add vanilla. Cool on stove for 20 minutes. Using a kitchen funnel, pour into a serving container. Refrigerate.

This syrup is not only a great flavoring for hot teas, but it mixes well with cold teas and lemonades.

Make your own vanilla chai by adding it to the chai recipe on page 24!

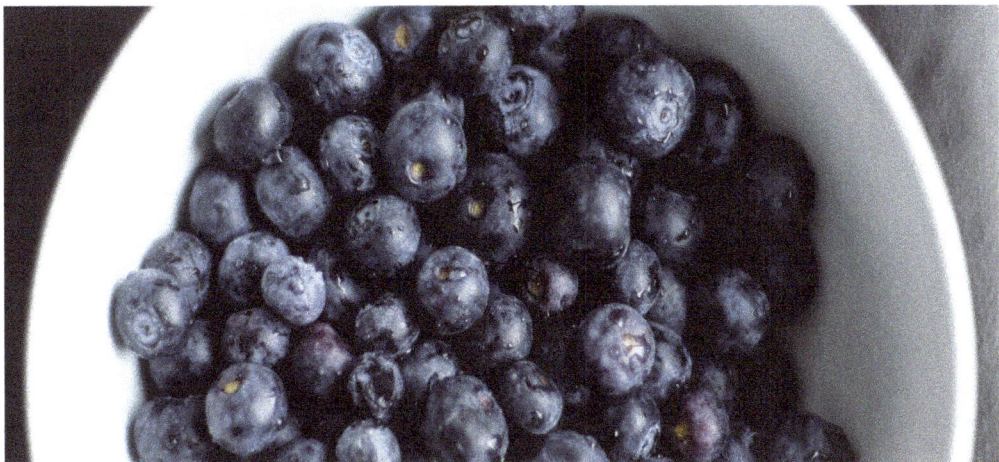

# Blueberry Syrup

1 cup water
1 cup blueberries
1/2 cup sugar

Yield: approx 2 cups

In a medium saucepan, combine ingredients and bring to a boil while stirring. Reduce heat and simmer until liquid is reduced by half. Remove from heat and cool completely. Using a kitchen funnel, pour into a serving container. Refrigerate.

If the syrup is too thin, you can simmer it a little longer to reduce the water content.

Add this syrup to the lemonades in the section starting on page 77.

# Herbal Index

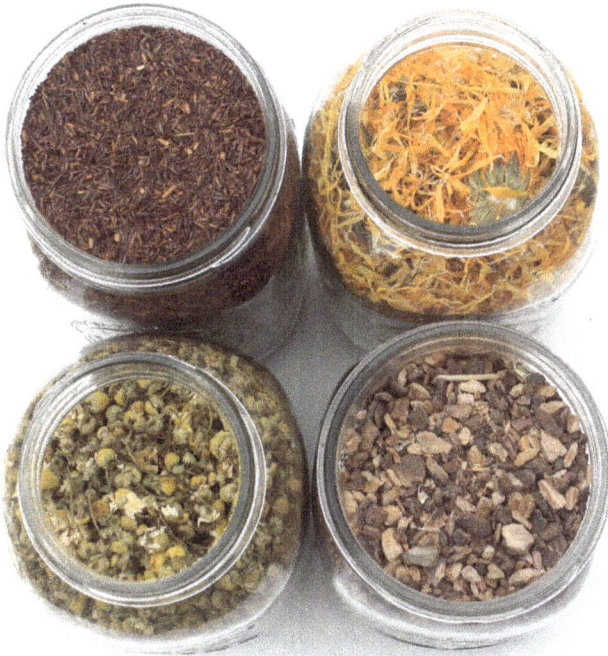

The following herbal drawings are for illustration purposes only. Before wildcrafting or growing your own herbs, please consult an herbalist or your supplier regarding the correct species. The descriptions are of traditional uses and for informational purposes only. Please consult your herbal supplier for more information.

# Alfalfa

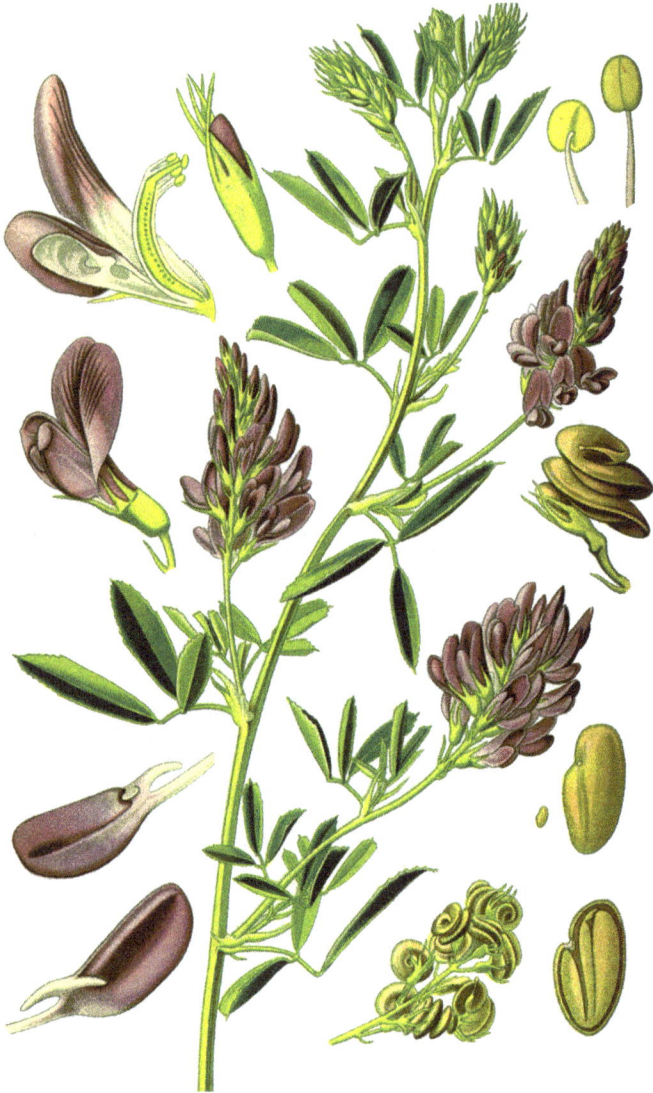

Alfalfa is a great herb for tea because it is high in vitamins. It has also been used for digestion and overall health. It is also said to have antiviral properties. Alfalfa's vitamin K content makes it good to use after antibiotics.

** Do not use GMO alfalfa since its safety continues to be questioned. Excessive use of alfalfa may cause photosensitivity.**

# Anise

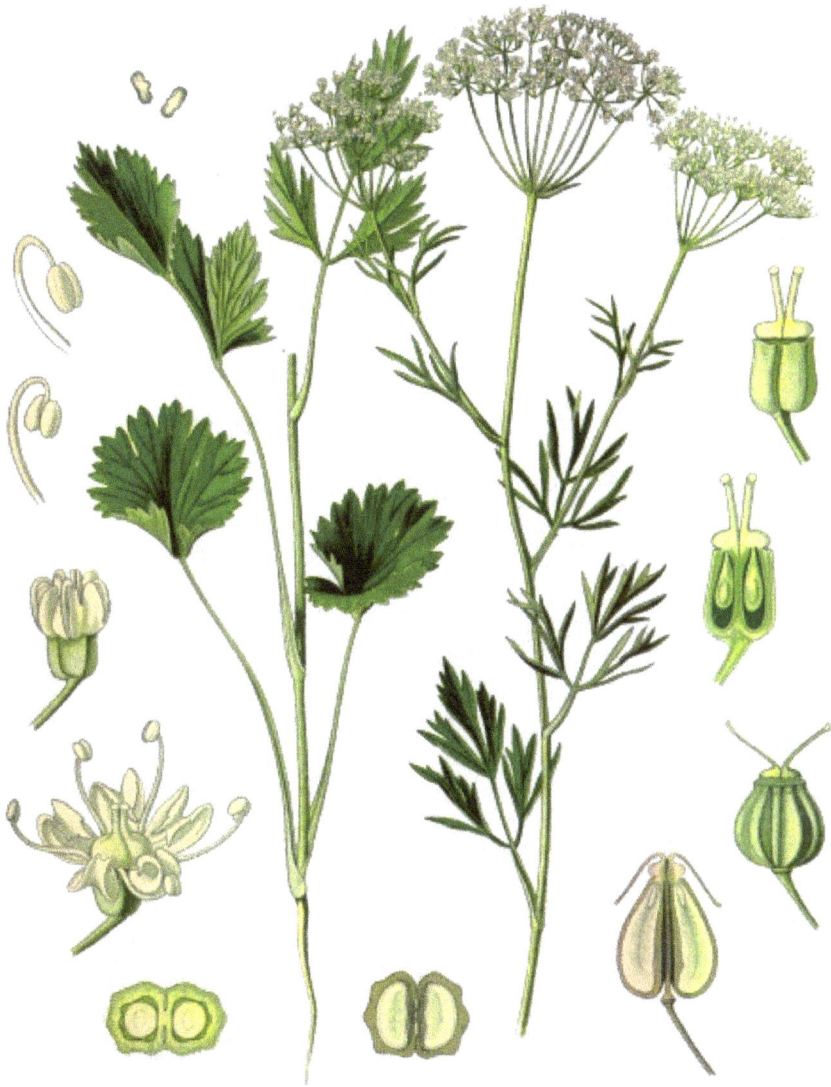

Anise not only tastes very similar to fennel but is also good for the same things that fennel is good for when it comes to digestion; namely nausea, gas, reflux, and indigestion. It has also been used as an expectorant, for bad breath, and for skin conditions.

** It is not recommended that you boil the seeds for a long period of time because too much of the oil may cause nausea.**

# Astragalus

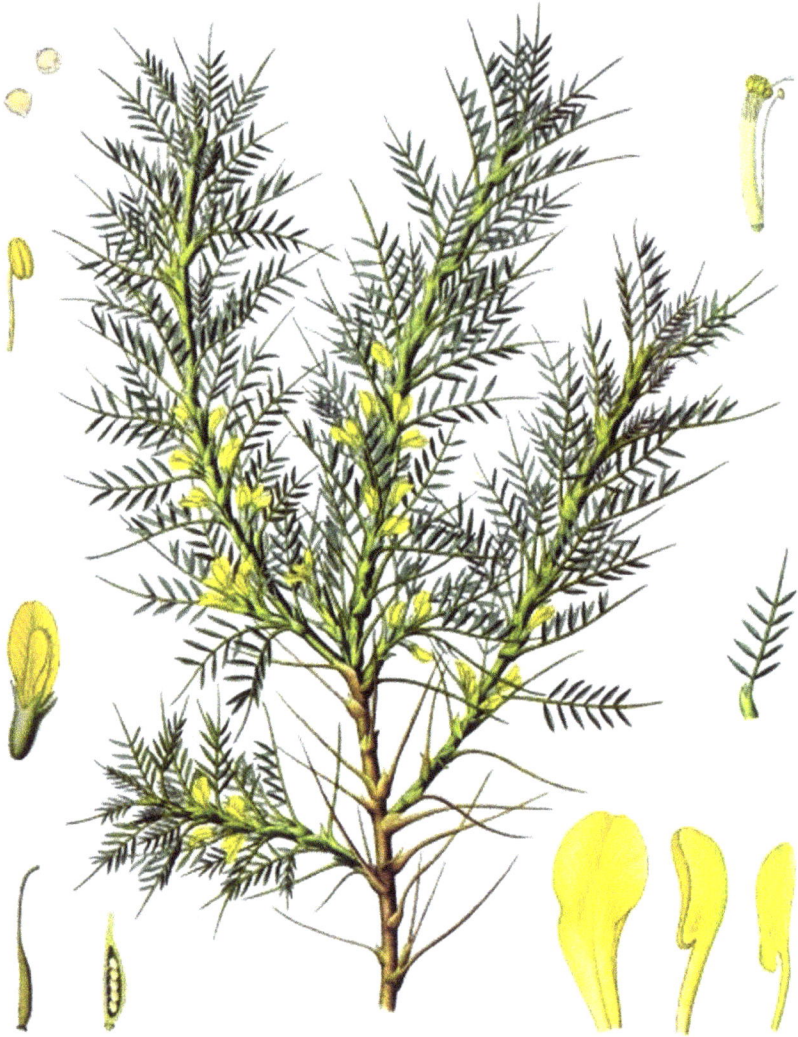

Astragalus root is an excellent immunity booster and a great herb to use at the beginning of cold and flu season. It is also said to be great for asthma and allergies.

✸✸ If you are suffering from an acute infection, or have an autoimmune disease, consult your health care professional before using. ✸✸

# Basil

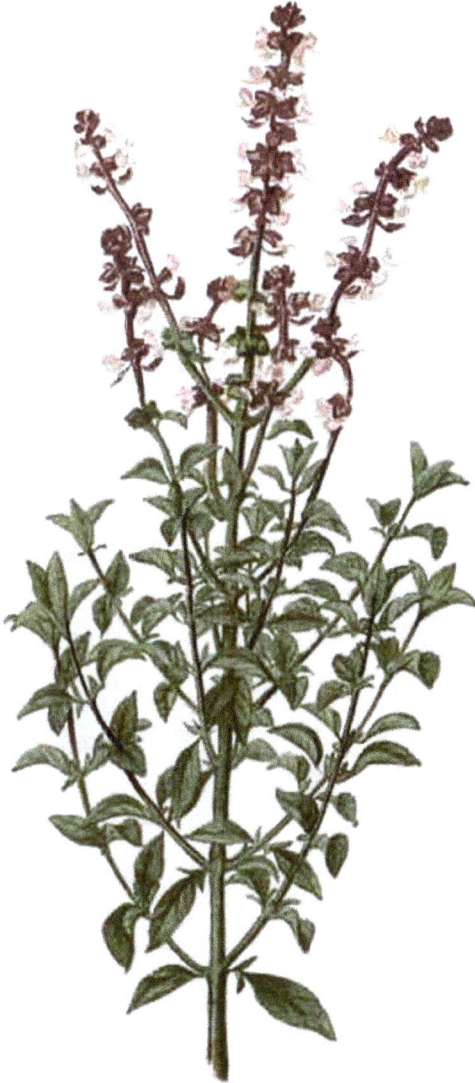

Basil has not only been used as an immune stimulant but it has also been used to relieve digestive complaints such as gas, nausea, constipation and indigestion. It is also said to help clear up acne and relieve headaches.

# Calendula

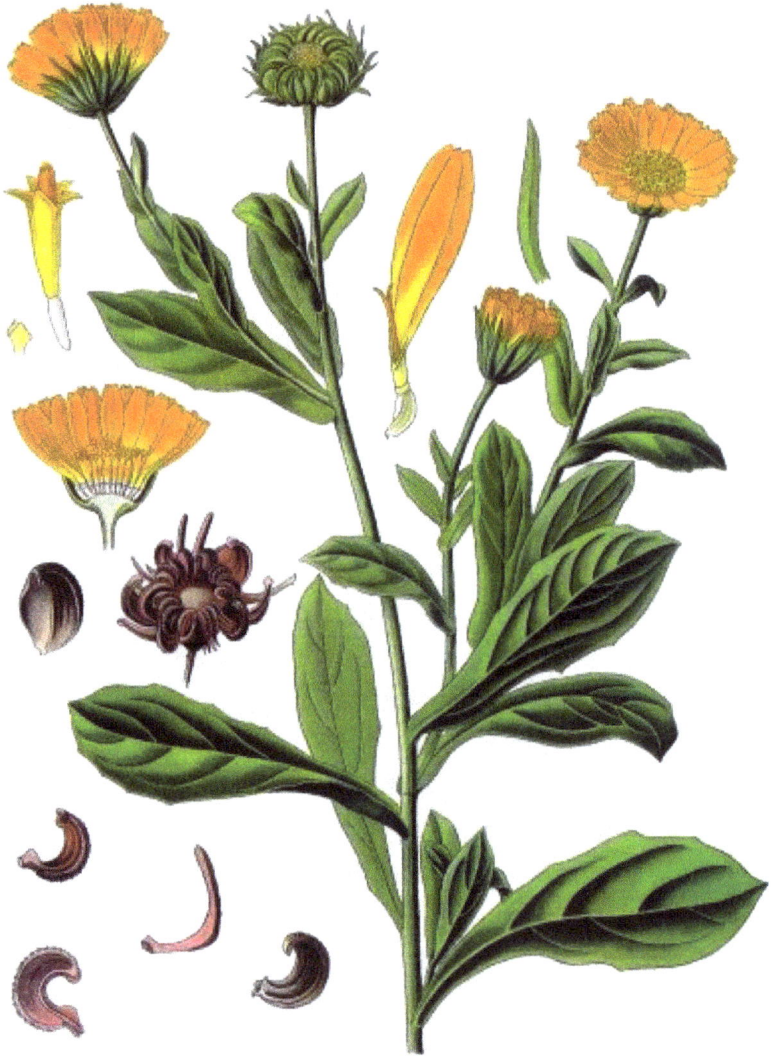

Calendula, also called 'pot marigold,' has been used for many external complaints but it has also been used internally for a variety of symptoms such as cough, indigestion, sore mouth and throat, diarrhea, fevers, and even acne.

** Those that have a hay fever allergy should try a small dose at first to be sure there is no allergic reaction. This is not the same marigold as the ones you buy for your garden so be sure you are using the right plant! **

# Catnip

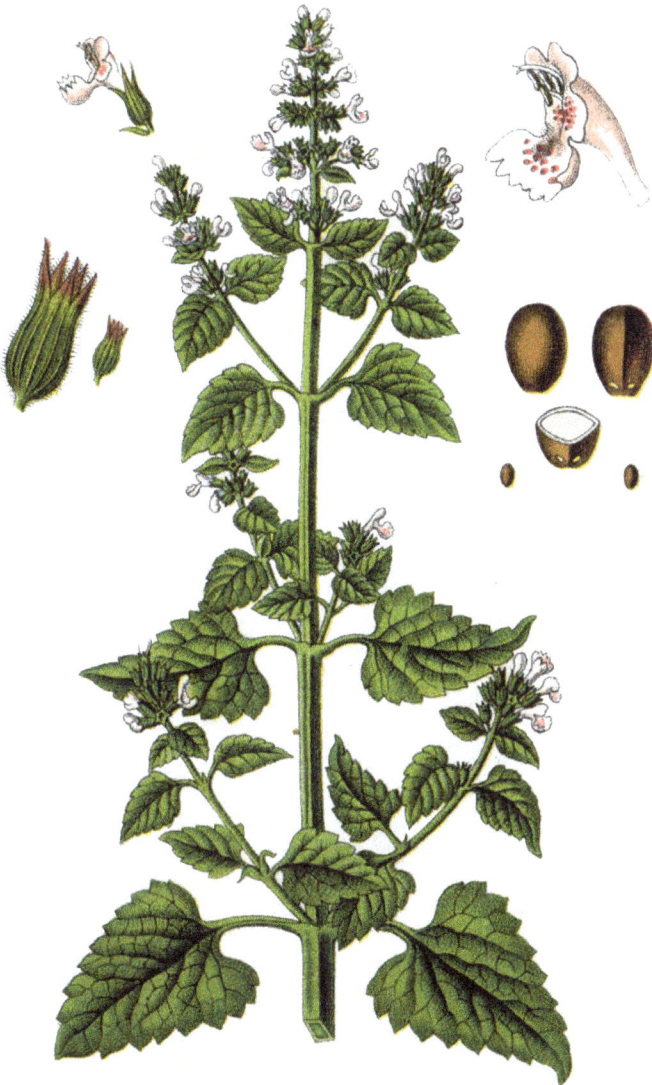

Catnip, also called catmint, is great for anxiety or nervousness because it has the same chemical in it as valerian. Because of this muscle relaxing chemical, it is also good for stomach complaints, headaches and diarrhea. It is especially great for colds and flu because of its ability to rid the body of toxins through sweat as well as relieving body aches that can be associated with the cold and flu. This herb is a diuretic so you may not want to use it too close to bedtime.

# Chamomile

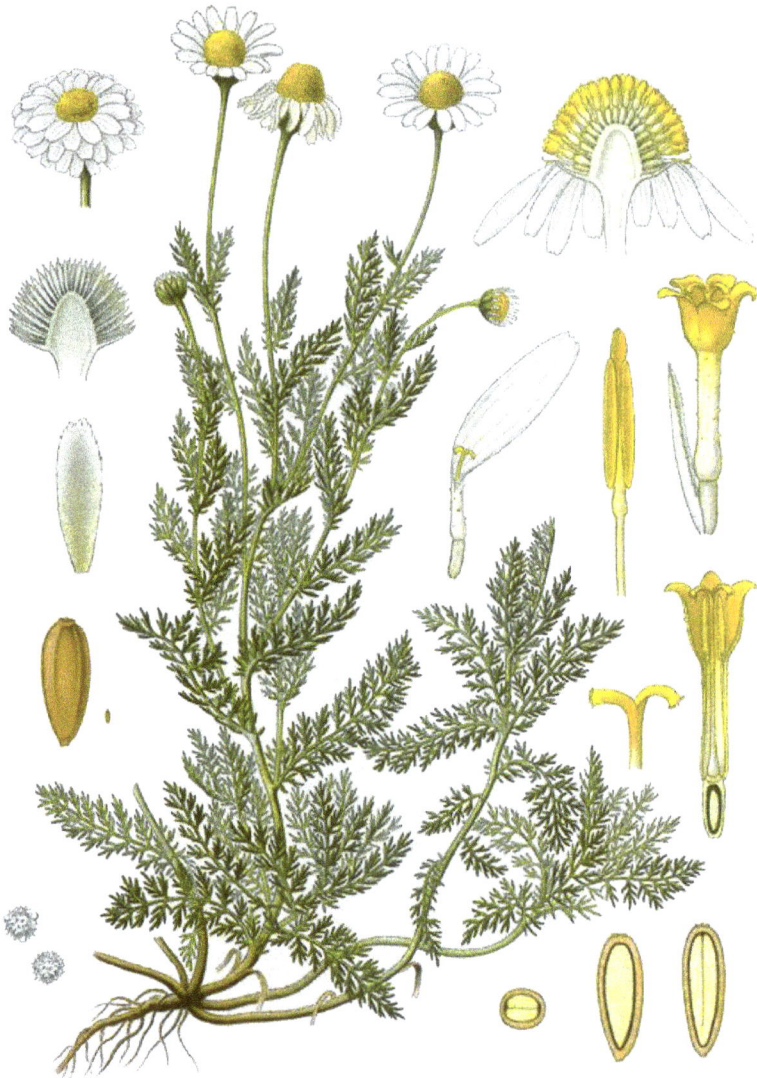

Chamomile is a relaxing herb that is great for anxiety and tension. It also can help with a lot of stomach and digestive ailments. Brewed as a strong tea, it can be used as a mouthwash for mouth irritations. This herb is a diuretic so you may not want to use it too close to bedtime.
❀❀ Due to its blood thinning affects, consult your health care professional if you are having surgery. Although rare, those with hay fever may be allergic so use with caution ❀❀

# Cinnamon

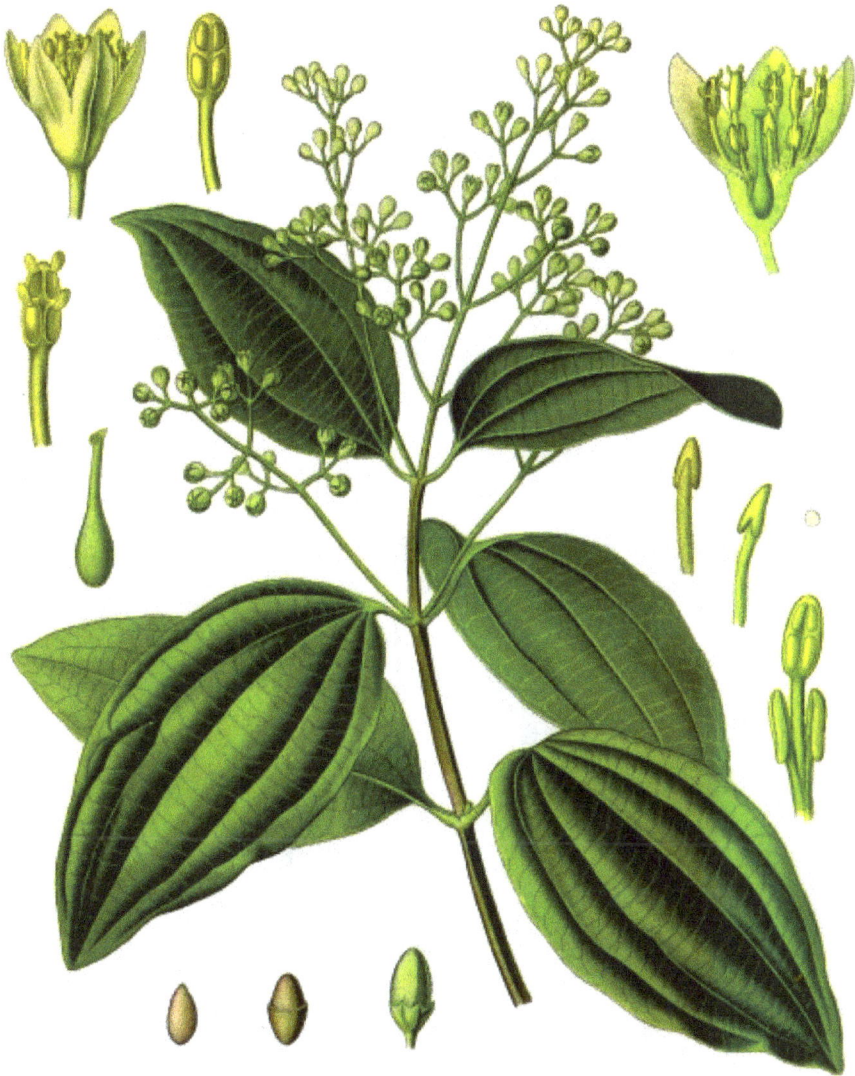

Cinnamon is high in antioxidants so it's a spice that is great for cold and flu. Due to its mild anti-inflammatory properties, it is also great for stomach complaints like indigestion, nausea, gas, and diarrhea.

# Cloves

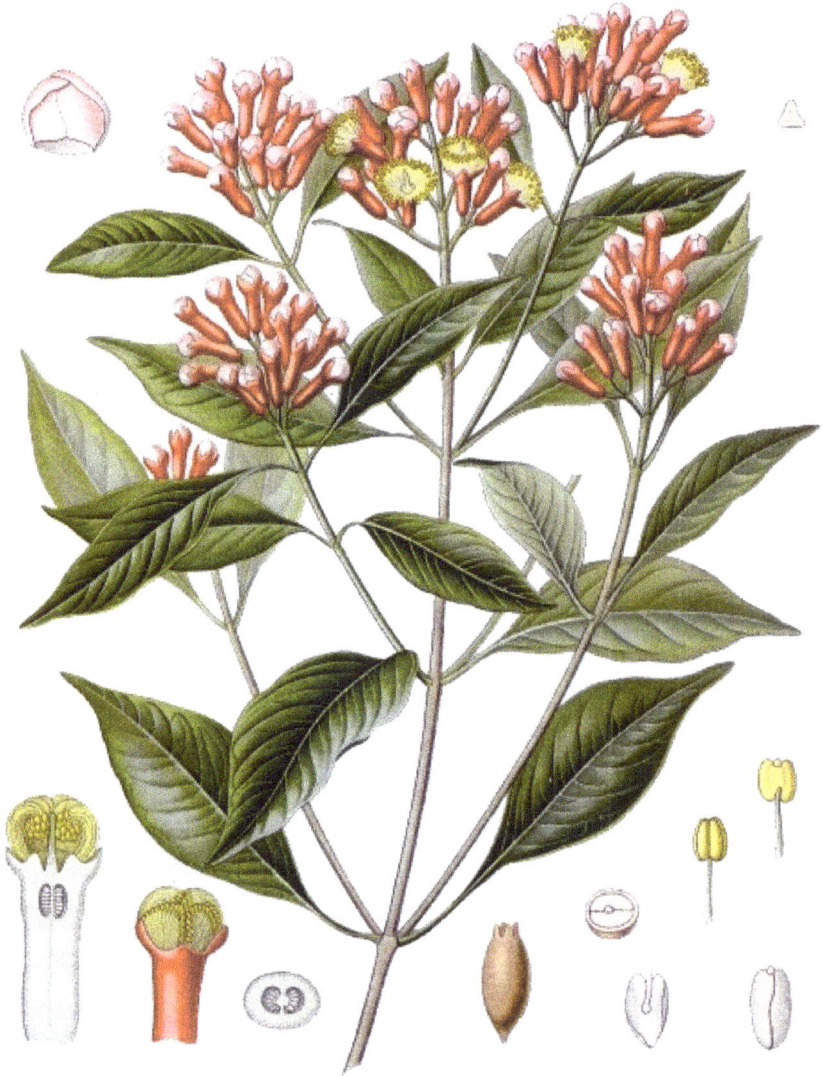

Cloves are a warm spice very similar to cinnamon and ginger and have been used as a similar remedy for digestive complaints such as gas, nausea, and indigestion. It has also been used for colds, cough, and mouth inflammations.

❋❋ For those with clotting or bleeding disorders, consult your health care professional before using.❋❋

# Cocao

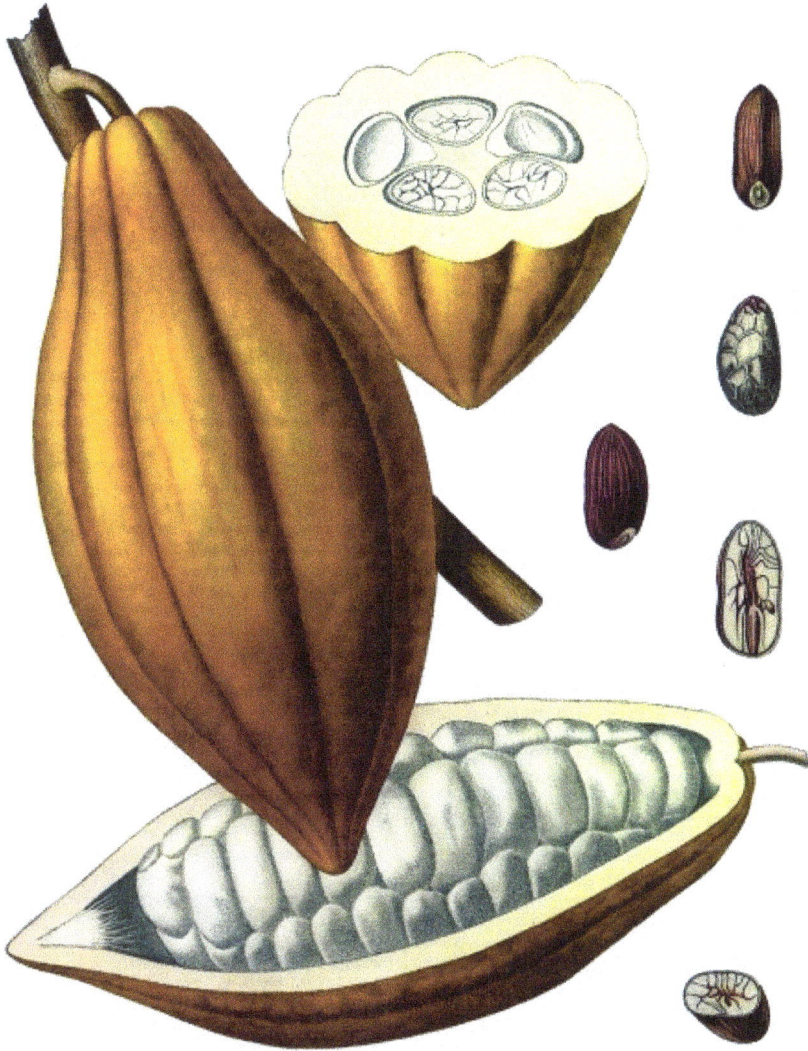

High in antioxidants, raw cacao's benefits to your health are still being uncovered. A single cup of cocoa made with raw cacao powder has triple the antioxidants as a cup of green tea.

# Cranberry

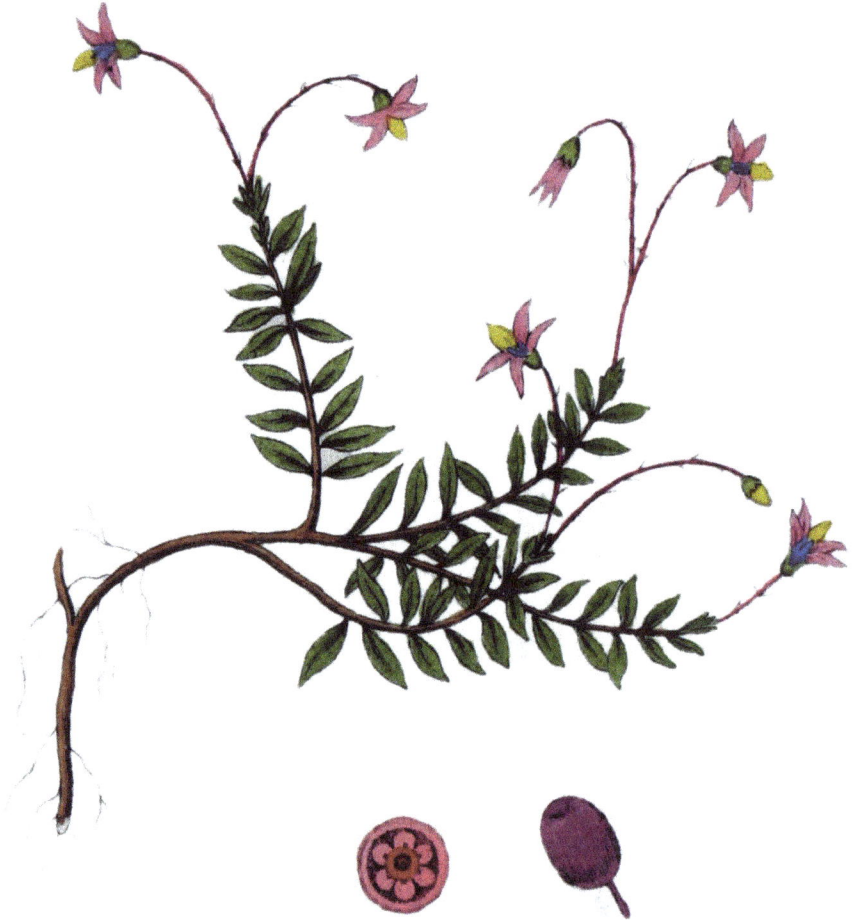

Cranberry has been clinically proven to help prevent urinary tract infections.

❋❋ If you suspect you already have an infection, please see your health care professional immediately. ❋❋

# Dandelion

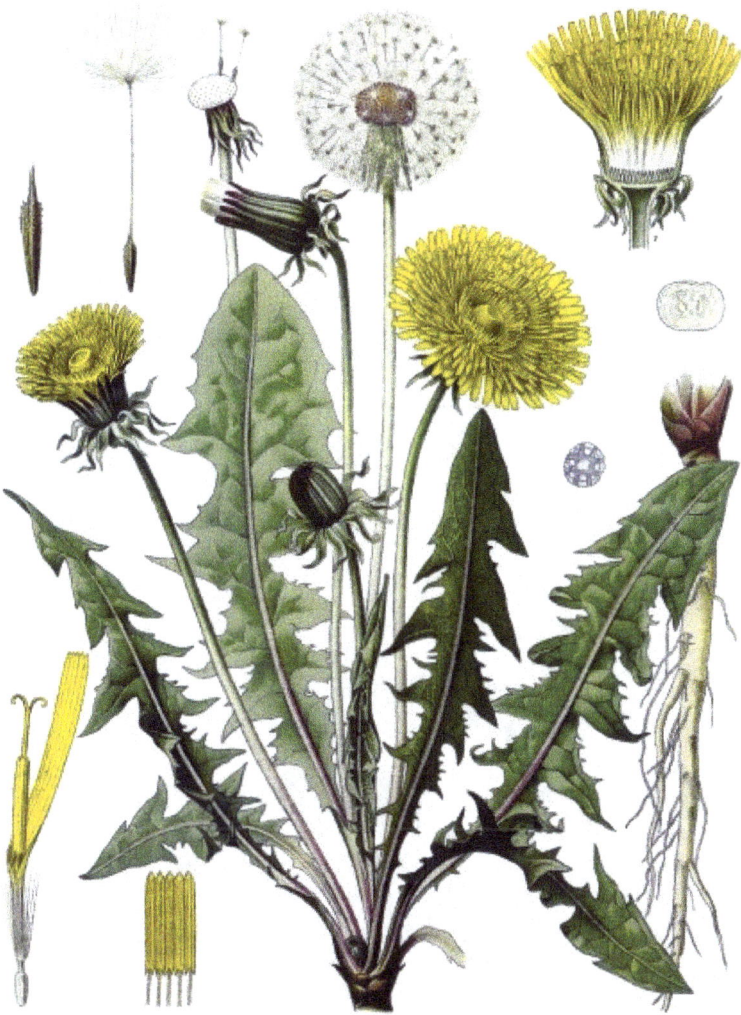

Dandelion flowers and leaves are edible as long as they are not treated with chemical fertilizers, herbicides, or pesticides. Best known for being a diuretic, dandelion is also great for clearing up acne and other skin conditions and is even said to have fat metabolizing properties. Its lecithin content aids in healthy brain function.

✣✣ Dandelion can lower blood sugar. Consult your health care professional if you are diabetic before using.✣✣

# Elderberry (Elder Flower)

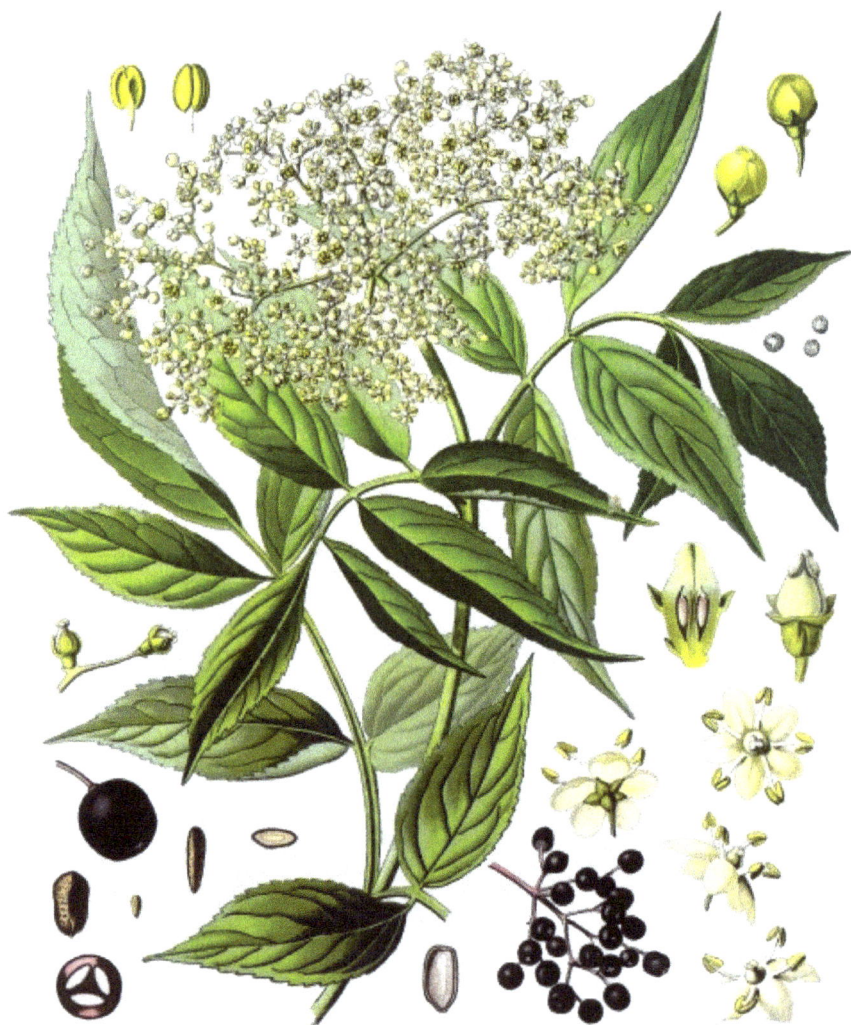

Did you know that elder is effective against 8 strains of the flu? Elder not only gives a great boost to the immune system but also helps your body get rid of colds, flu, and viruses that you may already have. It is also great for sore throats, upper respiratory complaints, and sinus problems.

** If harvesting, only eat ripe berries from the black elderberry plant. The unripe berries contain sambunigrin which is mildly toxic and can cause nausea. Boiling, baking or drying removes this substance**

# Fennel

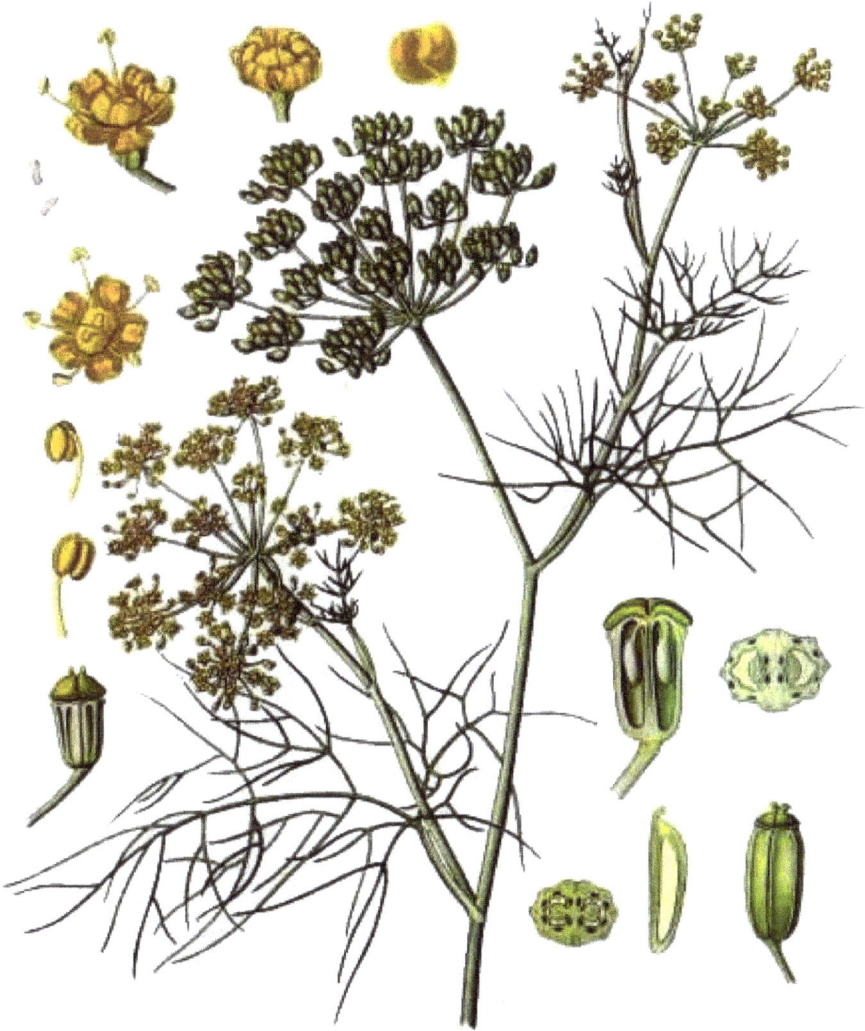

With a taste similar to anise, fennel is a great herb for digestion. It eases nausea, gas, reflux, and indigestion. It has also been used for hiccups, shortness of breath, coughs, sore joints, and sinus congestion. It has also been used for light sensitivity due to its high vitamin A content.

✻✻ If taking any seizure medication, do not use before consulting your health care professional. It is not recommended that you boil the seeds for very long because too much of the oil may cause nausea. ✻✻

# Garlic

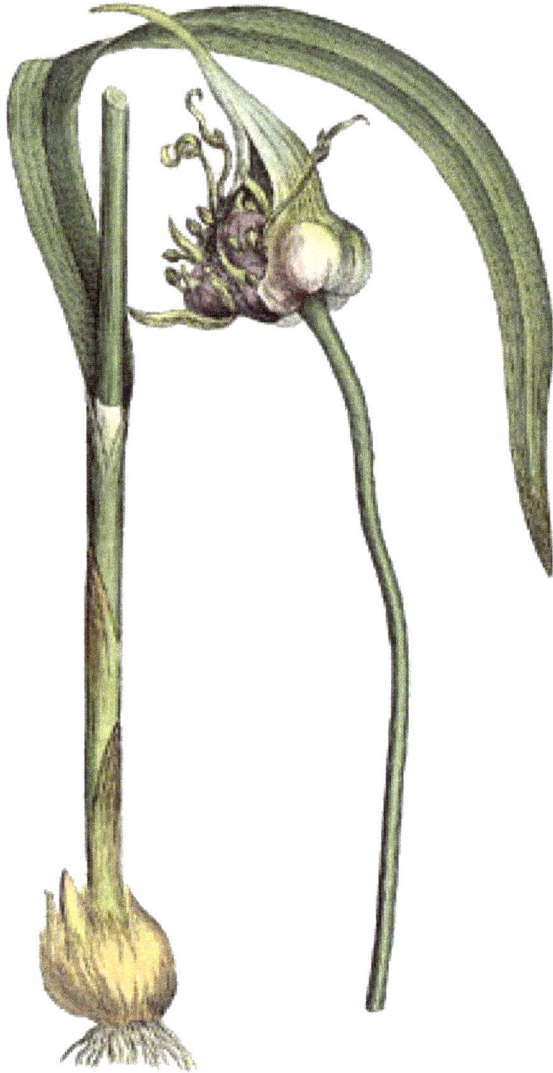

Garlic is not just great for your heart and cholesterol levels but it also boosts your immunity. It can also ease a cold, cough, and diarrhea.

** If taking anticoagulants, ask your health care professional how much garlic is safe for you to consume. Garlic can also interfere with certain HIV medications. **

# Ginger Root

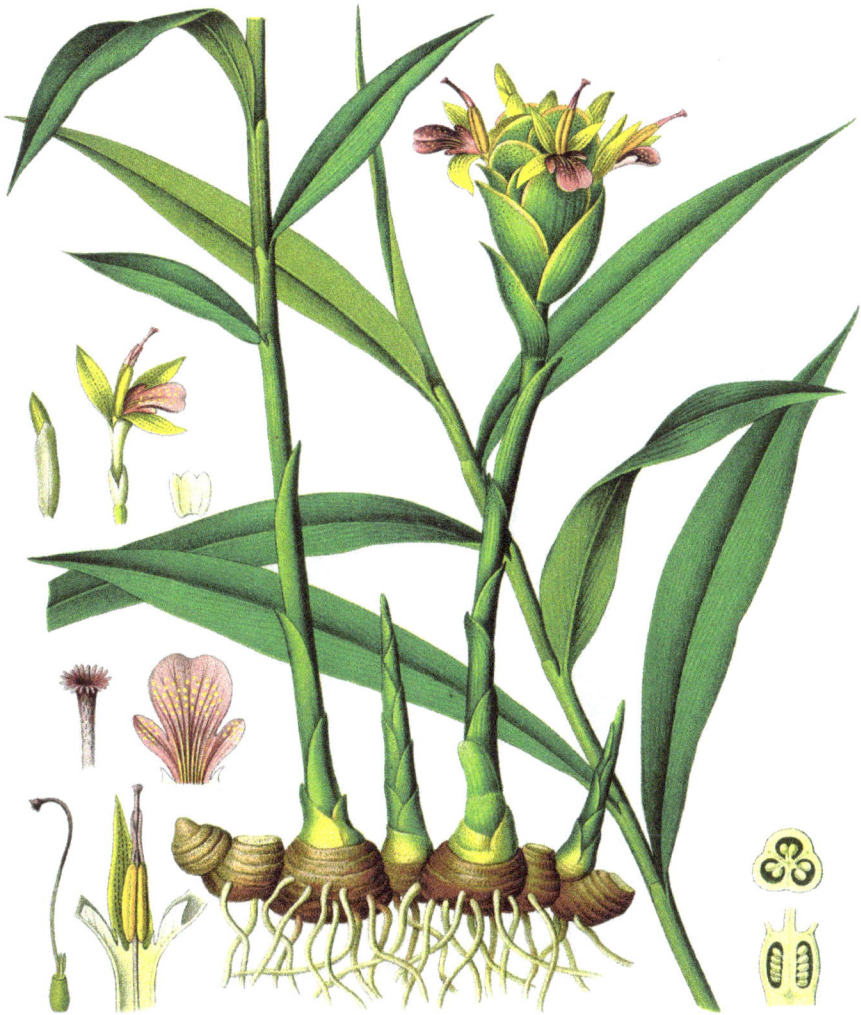

A favorite for travelers and pregnant women, ginger is the go-to herb for nausea since it neutralizes stomach acid. It's also a great herb to add to warm drinks when you are cold because it increases your circulation, especially to your hands and feet. As an antioxidant, it is also good for colds, flu, and coughs. It also promotes perspiration during fevers.

✲✲ May cause heartburn in sensitive individuals. Do not use during high fevers or if you have an inflammatory skin condition. ✲✲

# Hibiscus (use sabdariffa)

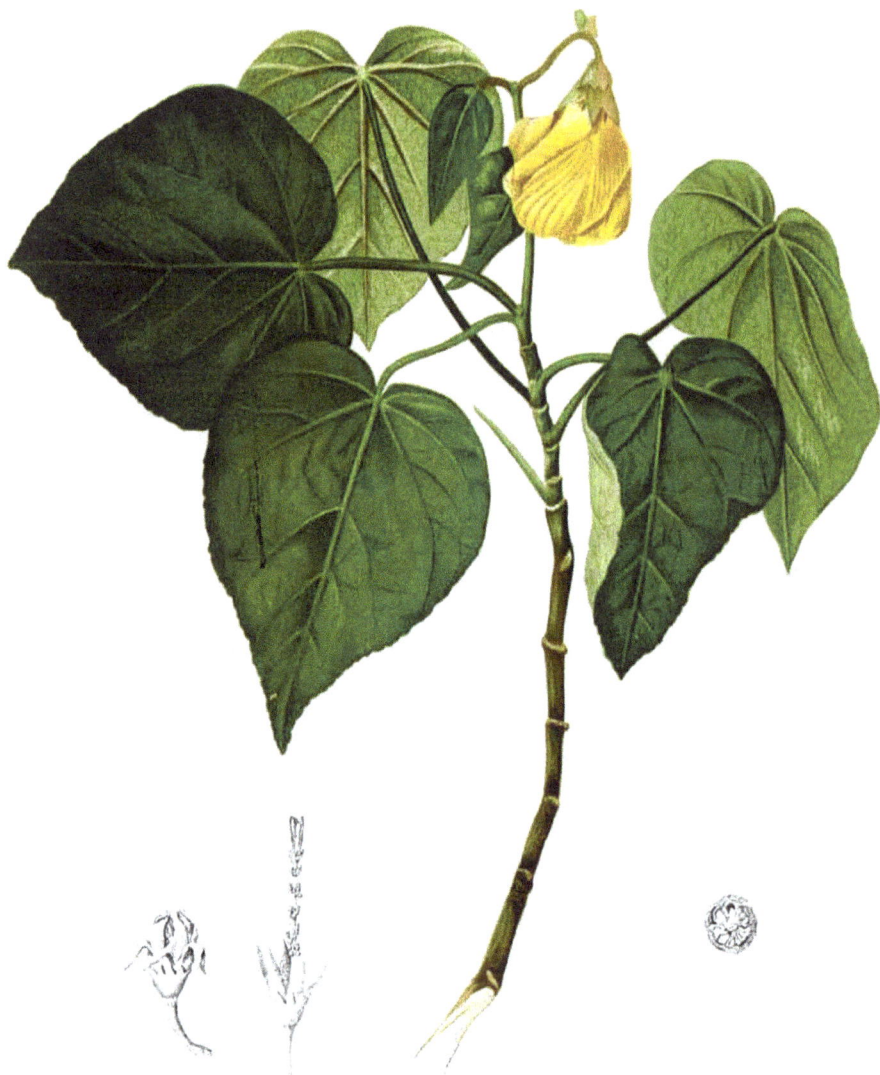

Hibiscus is rich in antioxidants as well as vitamin C. It can help promote blood circulation, lower fevers and can be mildly diuretic as well as mildly laxative. It has been used for colds and flu, sore throats, fevers, coughs, nausea, mouth irritations, and even loss of appetite.

✳✳ Make sure you use common red hibiscus, sabdariffa.✳✳

# Lemon Balm

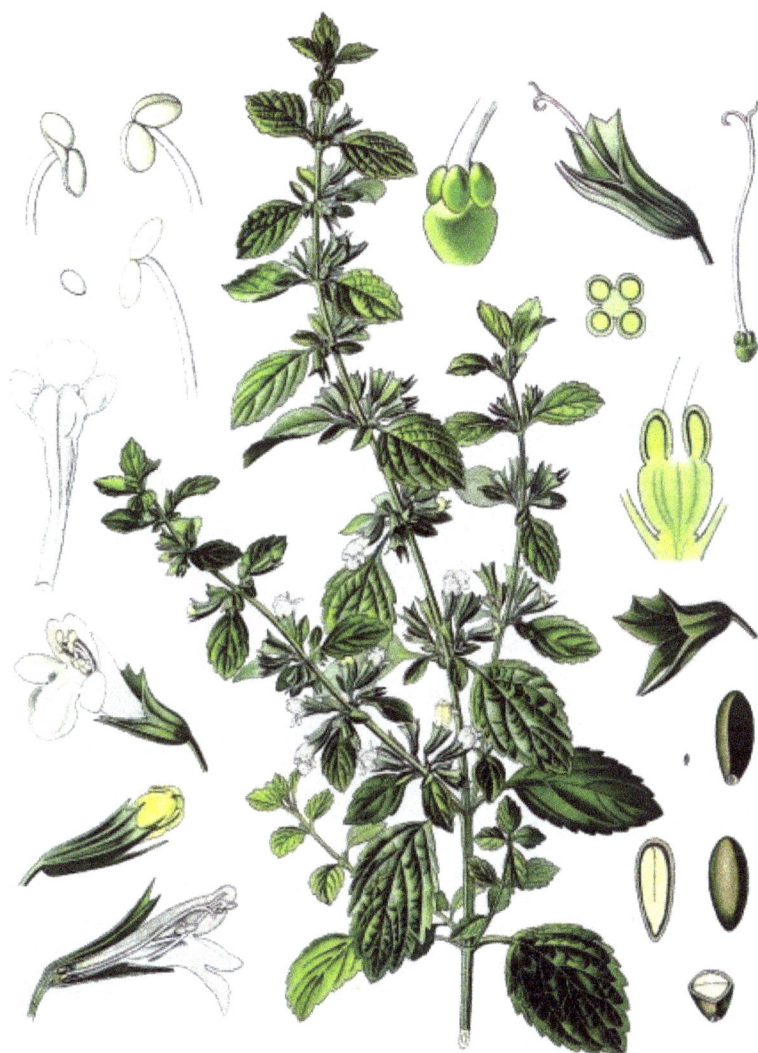

Lemon balm's mildly sedative properties have made it an herb that has been used for insomnia, nervousness, stress, and aiding concentration. Due to its ability to soothe the nervous system, it has also been used for fevers, colds, coughs, and stomach complaints.

# Licorice Root

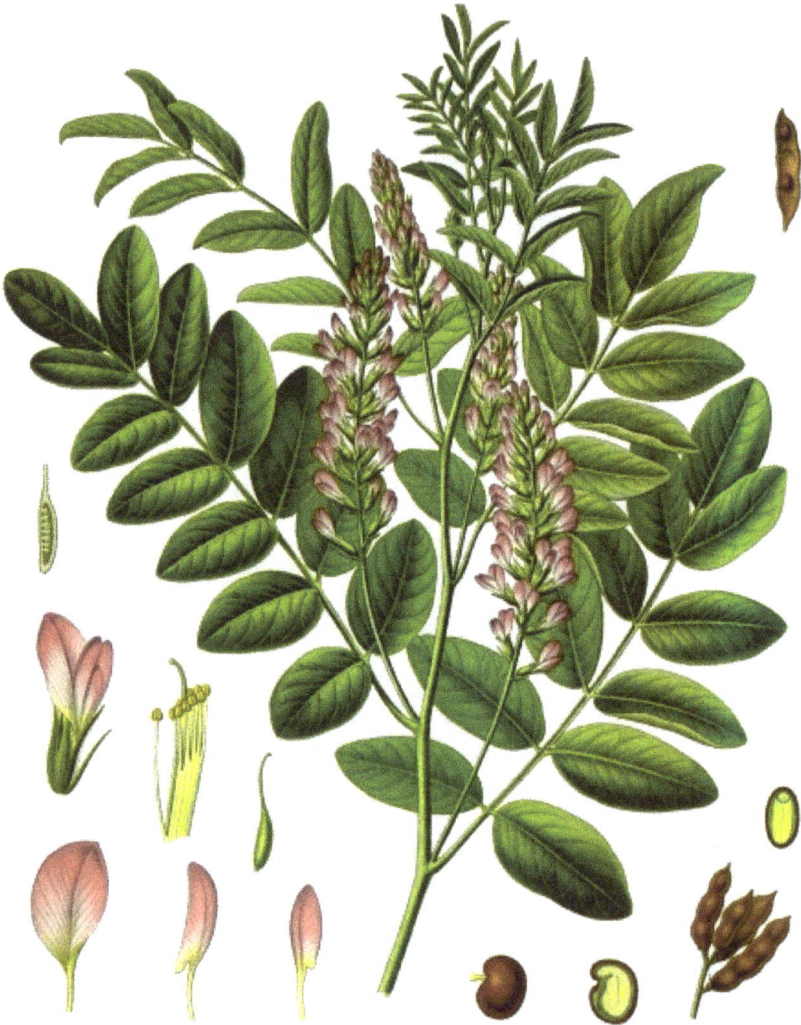

Licorice root (Glycyrrhiza glabra) is used for dry coughs, stomach aches, gas pains, and sore throats. Due to its similar properties, it is a great substitute for slippery elm bark. It is also a great addition to herbs that are strong or bitter tasting because it can mask those qualities.

** Do no take in high doses or for prolonged periods of time. It is not recommended for those on steroid therapy, have hypertension, are on heart medication or have bladder or kidney problems.**

# Marshmallow (HollyHocks)

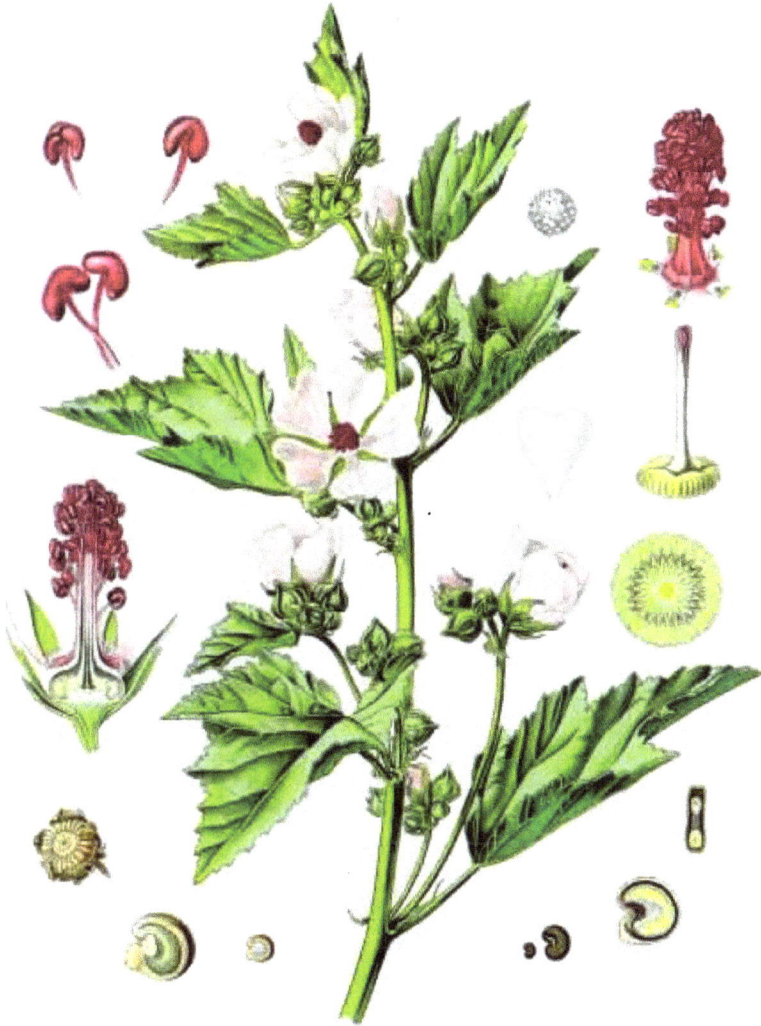

A great substitute for slippery elm bark, marshmallow has somewhat of a slippery when wet property to it. This makes it great for sore throats, reflux, and other stomach complaints. It is also said to be good for headaches and muscle aches. It is also a mild diuretic.

✸✸ Consult your health care professional before using if taking any medications.✸✸

# Mullein

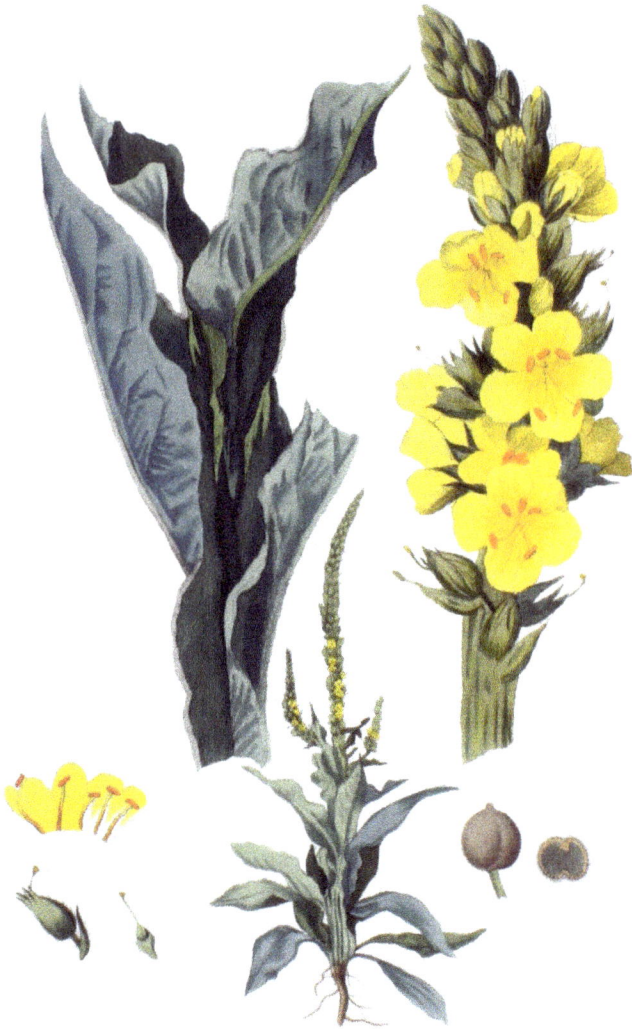

Due to its tissue coating properties, mullein is great for sore throats. Since it's said to be a cough expectorant and suppressant, it would be good for a dry irritating cough. Is has also been used for migraines and diarrhea.

** When brewing, carefully strain to remove plant hairs.
Do not use the seeds! They are toxic!**

# Nettles

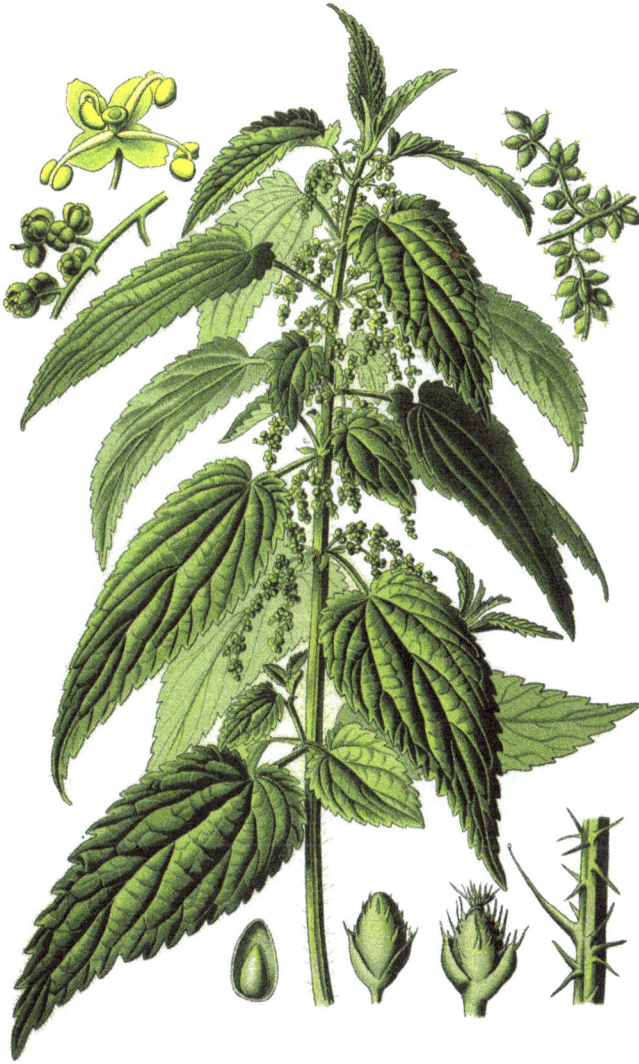

Nettles is an herb that is great for overall health because it is high in vitamins. It is said to relieve itchy, watery eyes caused by allergies. Several other conditions it is said to help are growing pains, eczema, asthma, and hay fever. It is especially helpful for healthy hair and skin. This herb is a diuretic so you may not want to use it too close to bedtime.

❊❊ Prolonged use can cause an electrolyte imbalance and can irritate the digestive tract. ❊❊

# Nutmeg

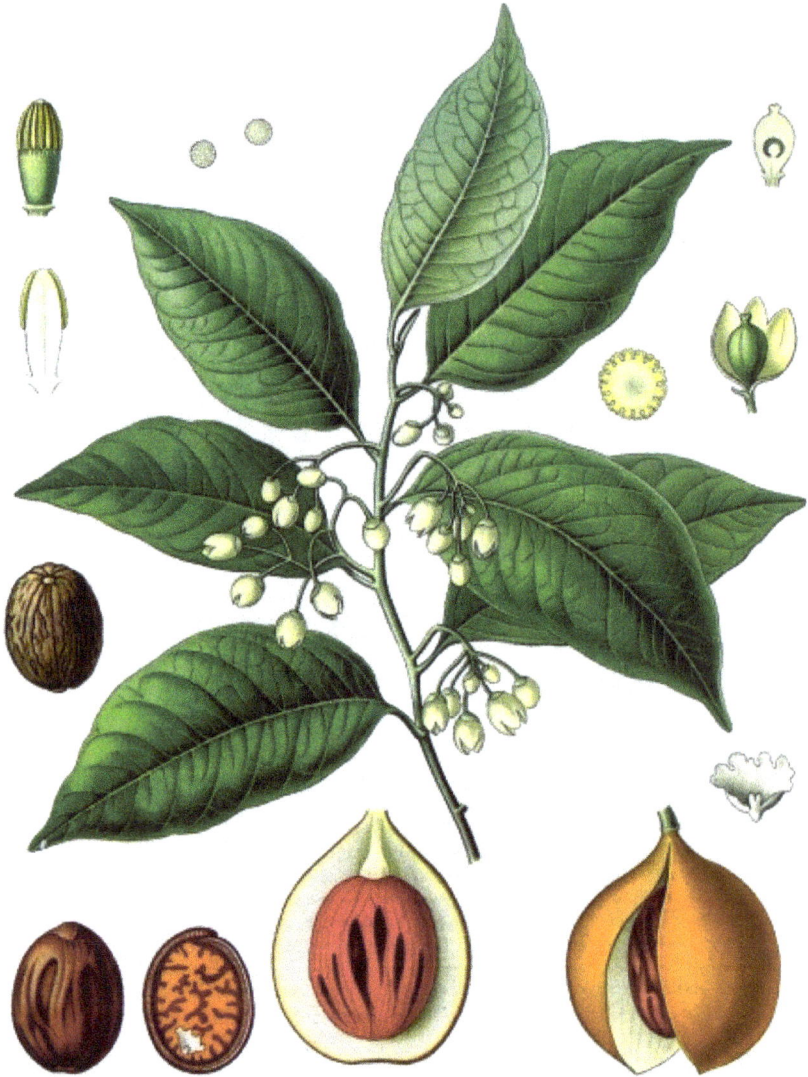

Another spice, like cinnamon, that is great for digestion. Since it is very strong, you only need a little. Great for gas, nausea, and diarrhea.

# Oatstraw

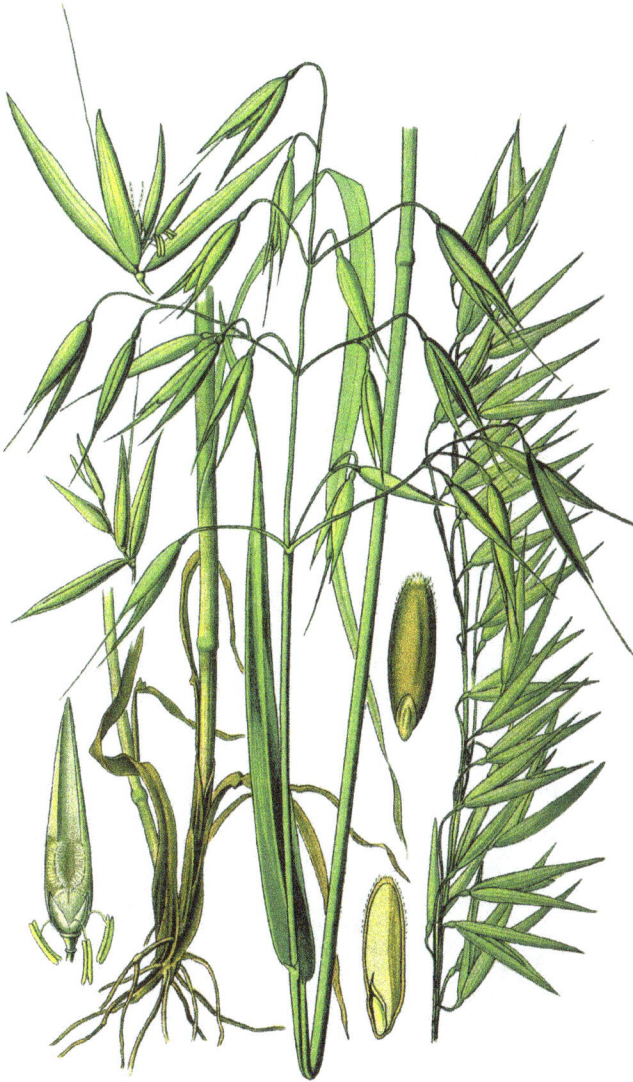

Oatstraw's calcium and magnesium content may help build strong bones. Its analgesic properties help ease leg cramps and growing pains. It is also said to aid your immune system, improve focus and attention span, give a mild energy boost, and help with healthy skin and hair. It has also been used for anxiety, depression and after illness.

** If you have a gluten sensitivity, use with caution.**

# Red Raspberry Leaf

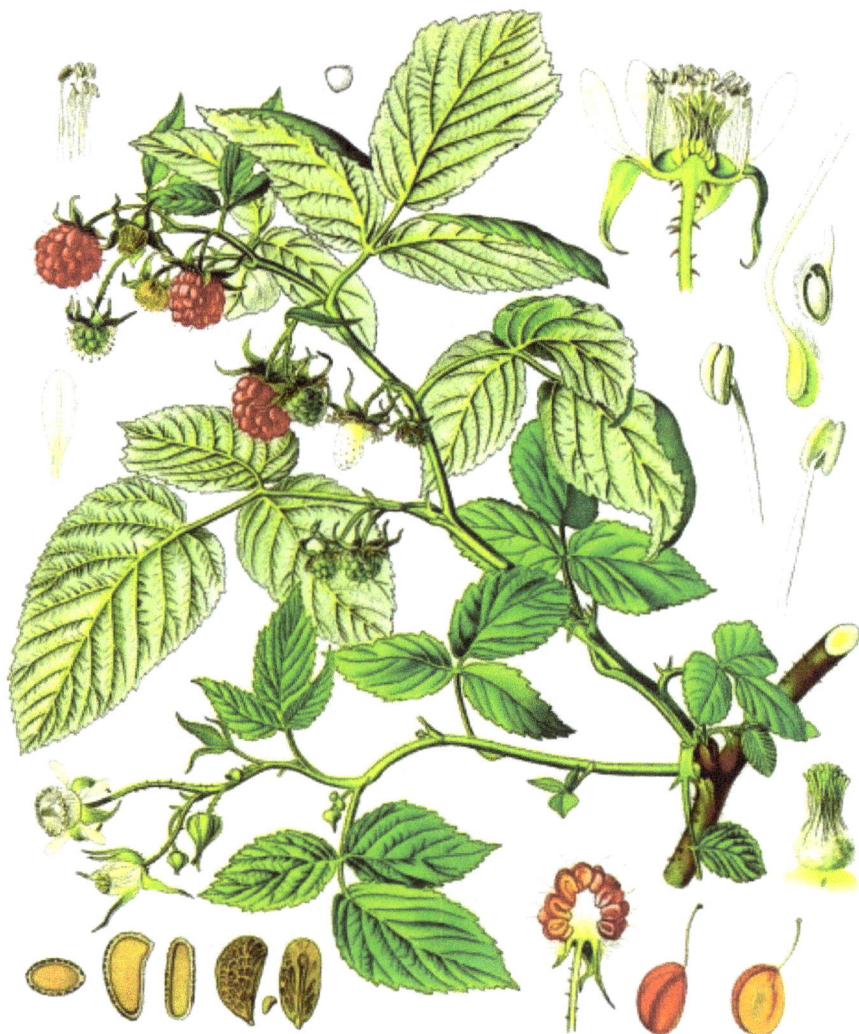

Red raspberry leaf is great for diarrhea, sore throats, and the tea can even be used as a mouthwash for mouth sores or other irritations. Its soothing properties are also helpful for stomach aches and as an energy boost after recovering from a cold or flu. It also contains a high amount of tannins which can be constipating so use in moderation.

** Red raspberry leaf may lower blood sugar. If you or your child is diabetic, please consult your health care professional before using. **

# Rose Hips

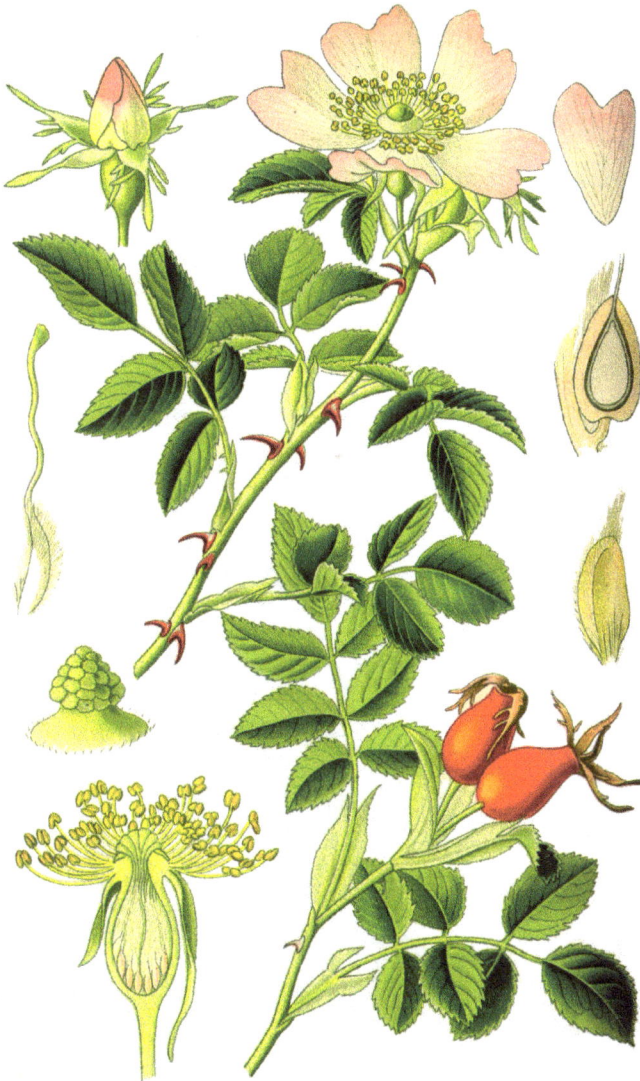

Rose hips are a great herbal antioxidant that is high in vitamin C. It is good for colds, flu, and normalizing digestion since it's good for relieving both diarrhea and constipation.

❊❊ Do not harvest this or any other herb that has been treated with pesticides or fungicides!❊❊

# Rosemary

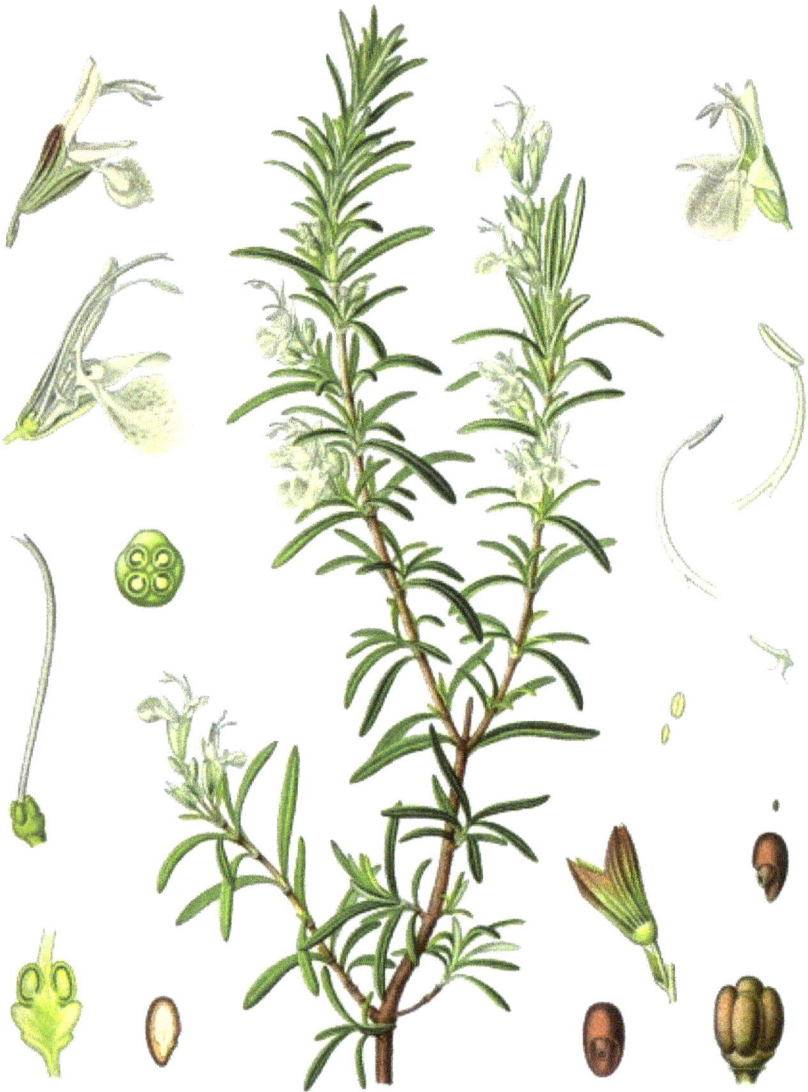

Rosemary has been used to soothe nerves, tension, and headaches.

** Can cause seizures in large doses **

# Spearmint

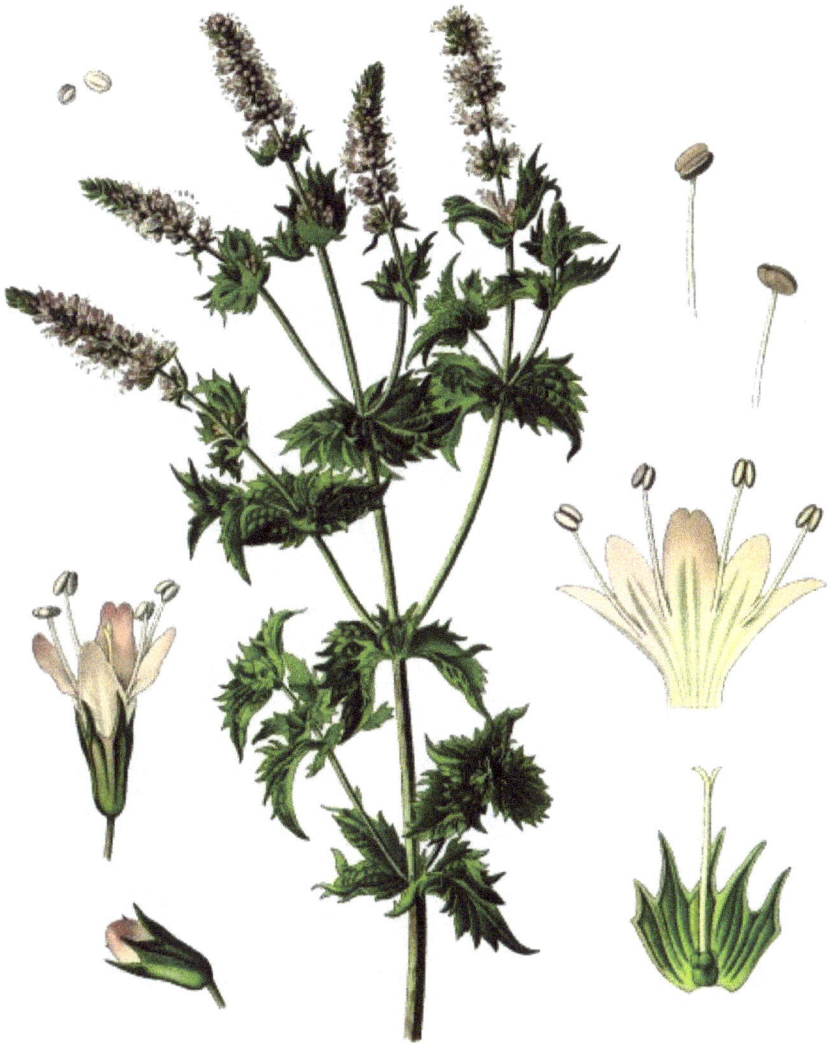

Spearmint is great for digestive complaints and is a great overall addition to almost any herb because of its taste. It is also great for colds, congestion, and headaches.

# Wild Cherry Bark

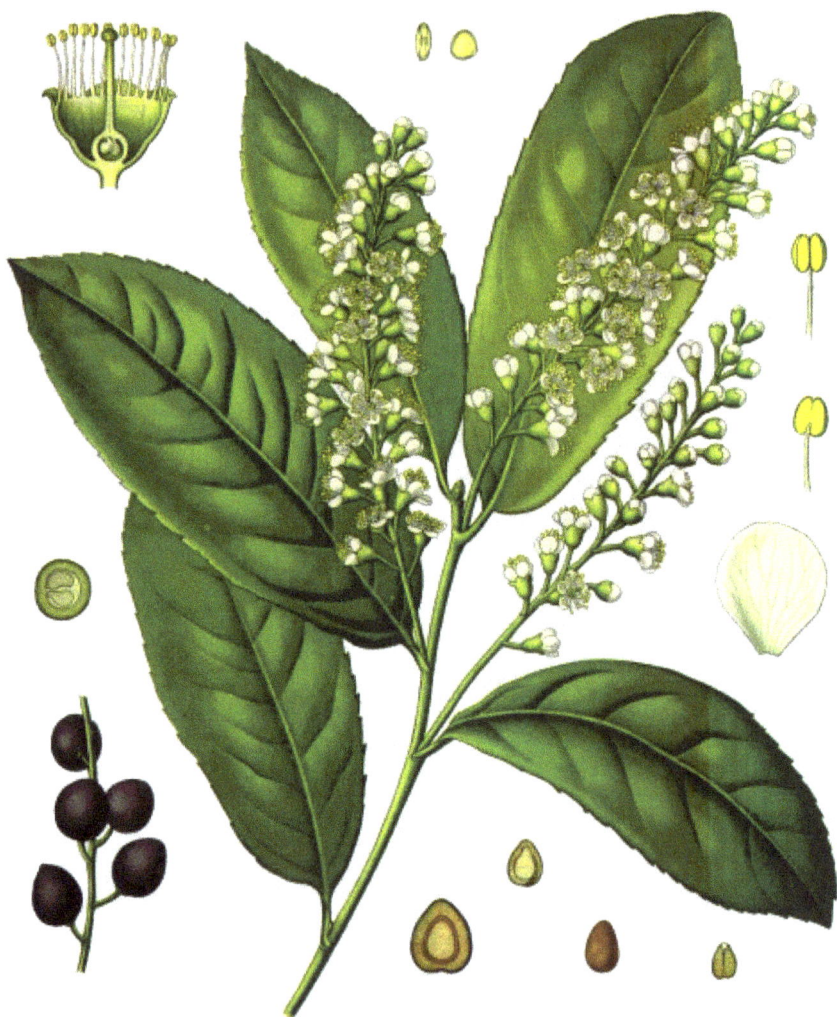

Wild cherry bark is a great herb for making your own cough syrup. It can be used for dry, irritating coughs and can soothe the sore throat that often accompanies those coughs. It is also said to have antiviral properties as well as the ability to help ease sinus congestion and diarrhea.

** It is not recommended to use wild cherry bark for more than a couple of weeks and not in high doses.
If using it to make a tea, only use 1 tsp per cup. **

# Harvesting Tips

**Astragalus** (root): In fall, after the plant fades - 4 year old plant

**Basil** (leaves): Harvest leaves once plant is 6 to 8 inches tall

**Calendula** (flowers): Half open blooms - mid-morning when dew has dried

**Catnip** (leaves): When blooming in summer and fall

**Chamomile** (flowers): When blooms are fully open - leave buds

**Cinnamon**: Cut branch - layer underneath bark is the layer you will dry out - use knife to cut strips off to dry - 3 year old plant

**Clove** (buds): When flower buds form - dry for 4 to 5 days

**Dandelion**: Untreated leaves and flowers in the spring - roots in fall

**Fennel** (seeds): Once flower heads are starting to dry

**Ginger** (rhizome): After bloom and leaves are fading, 10 months

**Hibiscus** (calyx): Once flower fades and outer leaves look shiny

**Lemon balm** (leaves): In the morning and when buds start to form

**Licorice** (root): Thickest horizontal roots from plants at least two years old

**Marshmallow** (leaves): After flowering (root): Late fall - 2 year old plants

**Mullein** (leaves): Youngest leaves in late spring/early summer

**Nettles** (leaves): Best when under 1 foot tall – wear gloves!

**Red Raspberry** (leaves): Spring- before the flowers emerge

**Rose Hips**: After first frost

**Rosemary** (fresh): Top 2 inches of 8 inch sprigs (to dry): After blooming, not more than ¼ of plant, up to 2 weeks before frost

# Quick Reference

**allergies** - nettles

**antiviral/flus and colds** - alfalfa, calendula, cayenne, cinnamon, elderberry, garlic, ginger, lemon balm, nettles, pomegranate, rose hips, rosemary, spearmint, wild cherry

**anxiety** - catnip, chamomile, lavender, oatstraw, rosemary, spearmint
    ~ see also insomnia

**congestion** - anise, catnip, cayenne, fennel, spearmint, wild cherry

**constipation** - cayenne, dandelion, fennel, hibiscus, licorice root, marshmallow, rose hips, thyme

**cough** - anise, calendula, clove, elderberry, fennel, garlic, ginger, hibiscus, lemon balm, licorice root, marshmallow, mullein, nettles, rosemary, spearmint, wild cherry

**diarrhea** - calendula, catnip, cinnamon, cocoa, marshmallow, nutmeg, red raspberry leaf, wild cherry

**fever** - calendula, catnip, cinnamon, elderberry, fennel, garlic, hibiscus, lemon balm, nettles, red raspberry leaf, rosemary, spearmint

**gas/digestion** - anise, catnip, chai, chamomile, cloves, fennel, ginger, lemon balm, marshmallow, mints, nutmeg, rosemary

**headache** - basil, catnip, hibiscus, marshmallow, mullein, rose hips, rosemary, spearmint

**insomnia** - anise, catnip, chamomile, lemon balm

**lethargy** - licorice root, oatstraw, red raspberry leaf, rose hips,  rosemary

**muscle aches/growing pains** - fennel, hibiscus, marshmallow, nettles, oatstraw

**post illness** - alfalfa, oatstraw, red raspberry leaf

**skin** - basil, calendula, dandelion, elderberry, nettles, oatstraw

**throat** - calendula, chamomile, elderberry, fennel, garlic, licorice root, marshmallow, mullein, red raspberry leaf, wild cherry

**urinary irritations** - cranberry, licorice, marshmallow

# Recipe Index

# Herbal Suppliers

Monterey Bay Spice Company
www.herbco.com
719 Swift Street Suite 62
Santa Cruz, CA 95060
800-500-6148


Starwest Botanicals
www.starwest-botanicals.com
11253 Trade Center Drive
Rancho Cordova, CA 95742
800-800-4372


Frontier Natural Products Co-op
www.frontiercoop.com
PO Box 299
3021 78th St.
Norway, IA 52318
800-550-6200


Mountain Rose Herbs
www.mountainroseherbs.com
PO Box 50220
Eugene, OR 97405
(800) 879-3337

# Further Reading

*Websites:*

**MedLine Plus** - https://medlineplus.gov/herbalmedicine.html
  • Wealth of info including health alerts and medicine interaction advisories

**National Center for Complementary and Integrative Health** - https://www.nccih.nih.gov/health/herbsataglance
  • Herbs at a glance as well as drug interactions

**Drug Information Online** - www.drugs.com
  • Searchable index of more than 24,000 prescription drugs, over-the-counter medicines & natural products as well as interactions

*Books:*

**National Geographic Guide to Medicinal Herbs : The World's Most Effective Healing Plants**
  by Rebecca L. Johnson, Steven Foster, and Tieraona Low Dog, National Geographic, 2010

**The New Healing Herbs: The Essential Guide to More Than 125 of Nature's Most Potent Herbal Remedies**
  by Michael Castleman, Rodale Inc, 2009

**Rosemary Gladstar's Herbal Recipes for Vibrant Health**
  by Rosemary Gladstar, Storey Publishing, LLC, 2008

**Herbs for Health and Healing: A Drug-Free Guide to Prevention and Cure**
  by Kathi Keville with Peter Korn, Rodale Press, Inc., 1996

**The Complete Illustrated Herbal**
  by David Hoffman, Element Books, 1996

# Immunity Boost Harvest Cider

This recipe is my take on Rosemary Gladstar's well-loved Fire Cider.
Use late summer harvested ingredients from your own garden and feel free to substitute with
what you have on hand.

1/8 cup chopped shallots or onions
1/8 cup chopped chives
2 - 8" sprigs of rosemary
1/8 cup sage
3 whole garlic cloves, chopped
2 Tbsp rose hips
2 hot peppers, chopped
raw apple cider vinegar
\* 2" piece of astragalus, broken or chopped (see pg 102)

Put all ingredients in a quart mason jar. Pour raw apple cider vinegar over ingredients to fill the rest of the jar. It's a little caustic on the metal lid so you may want to put a barrier between the lid and the liquid. Place in the fridge for *at least* a week, shaking daily. Most people usually leave it in the fridge for 4 weeks. After it has been brewing as long as you'd like, strain the liquid into another jar, pressing the liquid out of the solids. Store in the refrigerator. *To use*: Measure 1 or 2 Tbsp into a cup of hot water. Add raw honey and lemon, if desired.

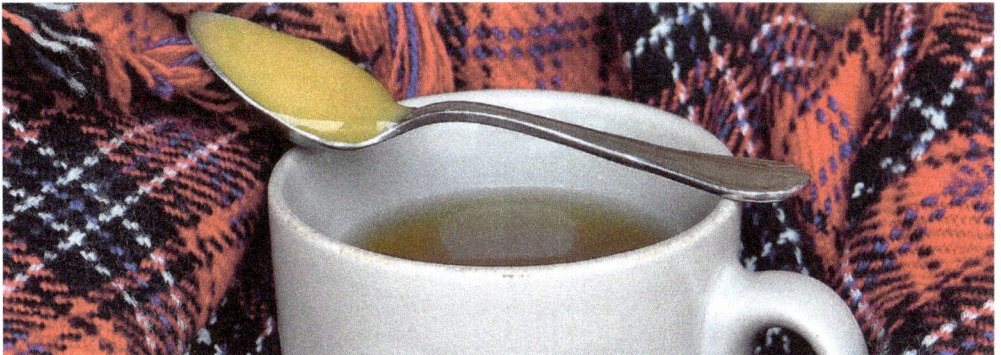

# About the Author

Robin Belliveau, ACC, ECPC is the author of **The Herbal Beverage Book**. In addition to being an herbalist, she is also a Certified Professional Coach who is passionate about helping people live healthy and fulfilling lives. She is a survivor of late diagnosed Lyme disease and has been an advocate for educating others about the disease. She lives in Massachusetts with her husband, four children, and three step children.

www.ingramcontent.com/pod-product-compliance
Lightning Source LLC
Chambersburg PA
CBHW072138020426
42334CB00018B/1848